Gerontological Social Work in Home Health Care

Gerontological Social Work in Home Health Care

Rose Dobrof, Editor

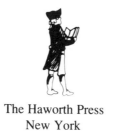

The Haworth Press
New York

Gerontological Social Work in Home Health Care has also been published as *Journal of Gerontological Social Work,* Volume 7, Number 4, July 1984.

The Haworth Press, Inc., 28 East 22 Street, New York, NY 10010

Library of Congress Cataloging in Publication Data
Main entry under title:

Gerontological social work in home health care.

Published also as v. 7, no. 4, July 1984 of the Journal of gerontological social work.
Includes bibliographies.
1. Social work with the aged—United States—Addresses, essays, lectures. 2. Home care services—United States—Addresses, essays, lectures. 3. Aged—Home care—United States—Addresses, essays, lectures. I. Dobrof, Rose.
HV1461.G47 1984   362.6   84-10924
ISBN 0-86656-337-7

Gerontological Social Work in Home Health Care

Journal of Gerontological Social Work
Volume 7, Number 4

CONTENTS

SHELDON TOBIN, PhD, *Director, Ringel Institute of Gerontology, Albany, NY*
TERESA JORDAN TUZIL, MSW, *Consultant on Aging, New York, NY*
EDNA WASSER, MSW, *Consultant, Fellow, Gerontological Society, Miami, FL*
MARY WYLIE, PhD, *Professor, Department of Social Work, University of Wisconsin, Madison, WI*

FROM THE EDITOR

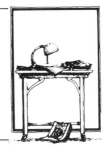

This is another in our series of volumes devoted to special topics; in this issue the focus of our attention is on service delivery and social work practice with vulnerable elderly and their families in the community. The range of programs described is instructive, providing evidence of the variety of settings and programmatic approaches to service. Three of the articles are written from the vantage point of the hospital social work services department staff, reflecting the critical importance of the general hospital as a location for service delivery, outside its walls, and beyond the time of in-patient care of the older person.

Haber's article, describing a program of work with Black caregivers, with eight churches in the District of Columbia serving as locations for the program, underscores the importance of "mediating structures" like churches in the service delivery system. The article by Calsyn and his associates is the report of a research project in which the effectiveness of various approaches to the task of visiting isolated elderly were compared. The "treatment recommendations" merit particularly careful attention by administrators and practitioners.

Although Seltzer and her associates are appropriately cautious in presenting findings from the first year of a three year project, they are able to report a successful beginning at the engagement of families in the case-management role, and this project should yield very interesting additional findings about this important approach to service delivery.

The article by Frenkel et al. is of a different order: she and her co-authors studied the evolution of a day care program for older people, a program located at a State Psychiatric Center. The program changed as staff worked at meeting the needs of a heterogeneous group of older people, and with limited staff available to provide the needed services.

Finally, is the article by Nancy B. Ellis, who is a member of the staff of the Center for the Study of Aging at the University of Pennsylvania, and who writes from her professional orientation of occupational therapy. Her definition of the role and tasks of occupational therapists in the delivery of services to "frail disabled elderly in the community" should add to the social worker's understanding of the importance of this profession. And her call for a team approach is a heartening one.

We hope that *Journal* readers will find this volume useful for service delivery and practice today, and also that it will provide some building blocks in our consideration of what home care services should look like in the years ahead.

Rose Dobrof
Editor

Sustaining Frail Disabled Elderly in the Community: An Innovative Approach to In-Home Services

Nancy B. Ellis, PhD, OTR/L

ABSTRACT. Description of a project to expand the capacity of the in-home services system in a metropolitan area to meet the needs of frail, disabled elderly in the community. Traditional medical practice, education of health care providers and societal attitudes are three major reasons we have failed to develop adequate community services to sustain healthful satisfying community living for the frail, disabled elderly. Cost effectiveness, efficiency and the degree to which the enhancement of in-home service staff skills and the expansion of specific health care services to clients improved the quality of the elders day-to-day living are examined.

INTRODUCTION

Aged individuals in our society should have access to the services necessary to help them maintain a healthful, safe, personally satisfying and relatively consistent style of living. As a society we are idealogically in accord with these concepts; however, it seems clear that we lack the humane and the economic commitments necessary to implement social policies and strategies to achieve these ends. This is especially true for the elderly living in the community who are disabled and/or frail. Elders who need services to help them meet the demands of daily living, especially those without families, frequently have no choice but to leave the community in order to receive the necessary care in an institutional setting. The long-term

Nancy B. Ellis, PhD, O.T.R./L is Associate Director for Education, Center for the Study of Aging, University of Pennsylvania, Philadelphia, PA 19104.

This project was supported by the Philadelphia Corporation for Aging In-Home Service Division, Alan Martell, Director.

3

care institution is a necessary component of a continuum of care for the frail disabled elderly just as is the acute hospital. A community based system of care is an equally necessary component in this continuum. There is a gap in available health care services between the acute care hospital and the long-term care institution. This hiatus in the continuum of care should concern all of us, particularly those involved in serving the elderly. There are approximately 25 million people over the age of 65 living in the United States. Fifty percent of this group have more than one chronic health problem and 60% of those over 75 years of age have impairments severe enough to limit performance of one or more major life tasks such as homemaking, work or daily self-care activities. We generally refer to this latter group as being the frail disabled elderly. These individuals are the ones at risk of being institutionalized unnecessarily when there is a lack of community based care.

It is estimated that there are between 5 and 6 million frail, disabled elderly who need community services in order to remain living in the community. While the number of institutional facilities providing long-term type of care to the debilitated elderly increased by 65% between 1963 and 1979, there has been only a modest increase in the community delivered care for the frail disabled elderly who need such services in order to continue living in the community (Levine, 1981). Currently in the United States we have one home health or homemaker aide per 5,000 aged individuals, whereas Great Britain has one aide per 750 elders and Sweden has one per 200. Furthermore, one aide per 100 individuals is the suggested ratio to meet the need for community delivered services (Butler, 1975, p. 142). Fully 80% of the care received by the elderly in the community is provided by family members.

There are three major reasons why we have not developed community services to sustain healthful, safe and satisfying community living for the frail disabled elderly. The reasons relate to traditional medical practice and evolving medical technology, education of health care providers and societal attitudes toward the aged and infirm.

Traditional Medical Practice

In analyzing why we have failed to develop a continuum of health care services for the elderly, Maddox (1980, pp. 501-520) suggests that our commitment to curing the patient outweighs and overshadows the value medical practitioners, and society as a whole, places on long-term, non-curative, types of care.

He asserts that the public commitment to improving medicine's diagnostic and curative armamentarium will continue to take precedence over non-curative concerns and that it is unlikely that public resources will be allocated to developing a system of supportive health care services for the aged. This is not to say that a continuum of care will not be developed. He predicts that supportive care services will continue to evolve in the same piece-meal fashion that has characterized their development in the United States to date. Current federal policies and allocation of resources seem to bear this out, thus increasing the importance of local initiatives to develop community based health care services for the frail disabled elderly. Such an initiative is described below in this report of a project to improve and to expand the in-home services component of an area agency on aging in a large metropolitan area.

In the United States, medical practice and research have traditionally been based on an acute illness, curative, model; a model clearly reflected in the educational process. This presents a problem for the field of aging in that the curative model is neither appropriate or applicable to the health care needs of the frail and disabled elderly. In medical education, commitment to this model has begun to change, but there is still considerable resistance to modifying medical and dental school curriculums to include material on normal aging processes, pathologies of aging and diagnosis and treatment of chronic disease and dysfunction.

Other health care disciplines, notably occupational therapy and physical therapy, include a strong emphasis on chronic disease and disability in their curriculums. However, even in these programs, there has been little emphasis on the normal processes of aging or on the particular needs of the frail aged individual.

Moreover, students in one health care profession are typically educated in isolation from students in other health care disciplines. Students may have an opportunity to work together during periods of clinical education, but frequently one discipline meets another for the first time when each enters practice as a qualified professional. This creates a problem because community based health care necessitates the collaborative effort of service providers, professional and non-professional, from several disciplines. Practitioners who have little knowledge of other disciplines and minimal experience working together are poorly prepared for community based practice. Both of these factors—curriculum content on aging and chronic disease and interdisciplinary collaboration—need to become part of the learning experience of health care professionals if we are to meet the growing need for community based support services.

Societal Attitudes Toward the Aged

Underlying and supporting this situation in health care is a public apathy towards the aged, particularly towards the elderly who are frail or disabled. Private groups like the Gray Panthers and the Older Women's League, federally legislated organizations like Area Agencies on Aging, and academic centers and institutes on aging, are helping to shape new attitudes toward the aged and aging in our society. Heightened awareness of elder citizens' situations and needs can have a significant impact on the priorities our society establishes for the development and delivery of health care services.

The following pages describe an experimental project involving the provision of health care services to frail disabled individuals living in the community. The project will be discussed in relationship to the issues of cost effectiveness, efficiency and the degree to which the new services improved the quality of the individual's day to day living.

PROJECT

In July 1980, the In-Home Services of the Philadelphia Corporation for Aging (PCA) initiated a project designed to serve frail, disabled elderly clients. The project was designed as a short-term staff training and service activity (Ellis & Martell, 1981). It was supported by an allocation of end-of-the-year unexpended funds. The idea was to use the expertise of health professionals, in this instance, occupational therapists, to expand and enhance services to the elderly living in the community.

Five occupational therapists were employed for periods ranging from five to nine months. Each was assigned to one of PCA's five service areas. The therapists were responsible to the coordinator of in-home services in their respective areas. The coordinator and the nurse consultant oriented the therapists to the in-home system. Working together, the coordinator, nurse and therapist identified the specific health care issues and needs the therapist should address. The therapists' primary responsibility was to augment and increase in-home and center staff's knowledge and skill in identifying and appropriately managing the day-to-day functional needs of frail and/or disabled elderly clients. Their secondary role was to provide occupational therapy services to elderly home-bound clients. Throughout the project they functioned in the dual capacity of trainers and service providers. To accomplish these objectives, they worked with in-home staff, senior center staff, nurse consultants, homemaker aides and elderly clients.

Approximately one hundred staff participated in a five month series of training sessions. The sessions included information on the functional deficits of conditions such as arthritis and stroke, on assessment of activities of daily living, on the use of adaptive equipment and on techniques of energy conservation. As a follow-up to their classroom training, staff members had the opportunity to observe and interact with the occupational therapist as the therapist assessed and treated clients in their homes. In addition, the occupational therapist worked individually with staff members consulting with them on specific clients and particular problems.

During the last three months of the project, in-home and center staff members referred over 200 frail disabled elderly clients to the five therapists for assessment and treatment. When the client's needs could be met on a short-term basis (one to three home visits), the project therapists provided the service. Whenever possible, they worked with the client's social support network (family, neighbor, homemaker aide) as well as with the client himself. They placed particular emphasis on modifying the environmental factors that could increase the client's ability to function independently, e.g., arranging living space for better accessibility via wheelchair. When the client's need for occupational therapy services could not be met on a short-term basis, the therapist made recommendations to the in-home staff who was managing the client's service plan about the type of treatment necessary and the community resources available to fill the needs.

FINDINGS

The introduction set forth three criteria for health care services to this population; namely, that the care provided should be humane, cost effective and efficient. Findings of the in-home occupational therapy project will be presented in these terms.

Humane Care

The basic assumption underlying this project is that it is highly desirable to maintain the elderly person, even those who are debilitated and disabled, in their own home/community setting. Clinical experience has demonstrated that elderly individuals will function best in the familiar surroundings of their own home. The therapists treated 189 in-home clients between February and May, 1981. Using functional assessments which required therapists to *observe* performance, 107 individuals were assessed as having improved in their ability to carry out self-care activities (personal hygiene, mobility, dressing, feeding) and to accomplish life maintenance tasks (household care, shopping, cooking, using telephone). Additionally, follow-up assessments by in-home staff demonstrated improvement in the area of leisure skills (use of time, self-expression, and need satisfaction). Seventy-two of the 189 clients maintained their current level of function. With chronic disease and its accompanying disability, maintenance of current functional capacity may actually be considered as positive gain. Without intervention to provide the client and his care takers with techniques for preserving function, conserving energy and adapting tasks to suit residual skills, the client's functional abilities would be expected to deteriorate.

The therapists each kept a written record of their daily activities and experiences. In the early weeks of the project, they made frequent notations questioning the appropriateness of the in-home services (meals, personal care, homemaker aide) for the clients they had had an opportunity to assess. It seemed to the therapists that in-home services were ordered for clients who had the potential to be independent. All that was needed was a short period of working with the client to show him how to manage for himself. The therapists were concerned that the client would become dependent on the in-home services. They anticipated that, over time, the client's competence and self-esteem would be diminished. Following the staff training sessions, this disparity between in-home staff and therapist assessments of the client's need disappeared. Staff's assessments and service plans demonstrated increased knowledge about the client's potential for function and increased skill in determining the appropriate choices in service planning.

Cost Effective Care

In the context of this project, cost effective care may be defined as the expenditure of the least amount of personnel time, energy and fiscal resources necessary to provide good quality service to meet client needs. In this context, it is axiomatic that the cost of providing community delivered service to the individual must be less than the cost of providing the same services in an institutional setting.

It was understood by all project participants, in-home staff and therapists alike, that the project was not designed to effect a decrease in services to the home-bound frail elderly. However, one of the byproducts of improved client function, particularly in the area of self-care skills, was a concomitant decrease in the amount of support service necessary to maintain clients in their present living situations. Within PCA the need for in-home services far outweighs their availability, thus any reduction in one client's services releases units of service for other clients' use.

Concern for cost effective service management was a central factor in the project's design. Over a period of five to six months, five occupational therapists helped to increase the skills of more than 100 in-home and senior center staff members. As a result, the staff were able to do more accurate initial assessments and re-evaluations, to identify the possibility of a client's functional improvement and to appreciate the importance of specific health care treatment to maintain the client's current level of function. The therapists were also able to add to the service manager's and the nurse consultant's information on rehabilitation resources in the community.

At the beginning of the project, some of the service managers expressed concern that being trained by, and working with, the occupational therapist would simply increase their work load. They felt it would cut down on the time they could spend on service management. With this concern in mind, the training sessions were scheduled into time already allocated to staff conferences and in-service education. Once the training sessions were completed, the service managers reported that they were able to handle the assessment process more rapidly, and with greater assurance, than before. They reported that they felt much more confident in completing the health status and environmental aspects of the assessment. Though no formal time study was done, these comments seem to indicate that training had the effect of increasing staff's skill and, thereby, the cost effectiveness of their services.

Efficient Care

Efficient care may be defined as the provision of necessary services expeditiously with as few appropriately qualified service providers as possible. In this context of community based services, the care provided must serve to enhance and/or to maintain the individual's ability to function as independently as possible.

The points made above in terms of the project's cost effectiveness also apply to the issue of efficient care. Specifically, the increased level of skill which the staff brings to bear in assessing the client and their increased knowledge about the resources available to meet identified needs.

One additional finding is particularly relevant to the provision of efficient care, that is the increased skill and confidence that family caretakers and homemaker aides reported as a result of the teaching the occupational therapists did during treatment sessions. For example, learning how to help a disabled person get from sitting to standing or how to transfer from bed to wheelchair can significantly decrease the time and energy expended in every day care. These techniques ease the stress and strain on the elderly client and the caretaker alike, conserving energy for other activities.

Another approach to gauging the effectiveness of the training program is to look at the project evaluations. Both staff and therapists responded to a questionnaire on the project. Comments from one of the service managers and one of the occupational therapists focus on the issue of effectiveness.

Service Manager

When I make a home visit I am now more acutely aware of the clients' environment, how they function within that environment, their physical problems and how these relate to the environment. Also when I record the clients' diseases and physical problems I am better able to see how they affect (or don't) a client's functioning. All of this helps me determine if the client is just unable to do a task (could benefit from adaptive equipment) or just lacks the knowledge to perform it. When writing my assessment and service plan all this information comes into play so that the service will be realistic to the needs of the client. (Ellis & Martell, 1981)

Occupational Therapist

The OT project has been most effective in upgrading the service manager's skills regarding medical diagnosis, functional independence and adaptive equipment. As the project progressed, service managers assessments reflected their increased knowledge by using homemaker hours more appropriately, using a greater variety of referrals. . . . The OT philosophy of promoting independence, rather than fostering dependence, filtered throughout the in-home services effecting the frame of reference of coordinators, service managers and homemakers. (Ellis & Martell, 1981)

These two paragraphs also serve to indicate the effect of interdisciplinary collaboration. The project demonstrates collaboration in providing community based care. In-home and center staffs are generally social workers by profession. Thus nurses, occupational therapists and social workers worked together to improve the scope, quality and efficiency of service to the infirm elderly.

DISCUSSION

The in-home services project generated observations and raised issues that merit comment here. In evaluating the project, perhaps the first question that should be asked is whether the community is, in fact, an appropriate setting for providing care to the frail, chronically disabled elderly. Could better quality, more cost effective care, be provided in some type of institutional setting? Clearly, there is no simple answer to this question. From the humanitarian perspective, community based care would be the preferred option because of the opportunity it affords to maintain contact with a familiar, physical and social milieu.

From the cost effective perspective, it is a matter of determining the point where the cost of delivery of services in the community is substantively greater than the cost of maintaining the individual in a setting where all services are grouped together. The difficulty of determining this break even point lies in deciding what factors to include in the equation of community vis-à-vis institutional cost. From the perspective of efficiency of care, here again, many factors must be considered. There is no generally accepted formula for measuring efficiency of care. Experience gained in this project generally supports the concept of community based care. One of the factors contributing to this conclusion is the observation that individuals generally demonstrate their best level of function in familiar environments where they feel comfortable. This precept has proved so useful that it has led geriatricians in Ireland and Great Britain to adopt a policy of carrying out initial assessments of elderly persons in their own homes except when acute illness necessitates immediate hospitalization.

Another factor that lends support to the provision of community based care for the frail disabled elderly is the availability of a large group of potential care givers—family, neighbors and concerned community agencies like religious groups and service clubs. These individuals usually provide care without a fee for service. Still another factor, yet to be empirically tested, is the impact of the community's expectations on the aged individual. The accepted social norm is that anyone living in the community will have an established pattern of daily self-care and life maintenance activities. By contrast, in an institutional setting, the social expectation is that the individual will not spontaneously demonstrate, or take responsibility for, his own activity pattern. This is not to say that all disabled frail elderly are more functional in the community than in the institutional setting. When independent function becomes too difficult, time consuming, laborious or painful to accomplish, or when community support systems are lacking, then institutional care is undoubtedly a necessary condition for survival. Under these circumstances, institutional care may foster an improved quality of life for the individual.

A second point in regard to community based care is the question of who should be involved in providing this type of service? Traditionally social services and medical/health care services have been delivered in the community by means of separate, essentially parallel, systems. There is obvious need for an interdisciplinary collaborative approach which capitalizes on the expertise of a variety of social service and health care providers. The problem is how to integrate and coordinate these services to provide ease of access and efficiency of effort within a framework of concern for the individual. The elder person's needs range from provision of home delivered meals and homemaking assistance to medication management and kidney dialysis. Individuals knowledgeable and skilled in specific disciplines are necessary to provide these services. At the very least, this suggests the necessity of close collaboration between social work, nursing and medicine. In the broader perspective, the range of the frail elderly's needs suggests that interdisciplinary collaboration among disciplines with particular skills in mental health, physical rehabilitation and legal and financial matters is highly desirable. The National Channeling demonstration project sites, all of which have medicare waivers, will provide data on the effect that a coordinated system of health and social services has on the frail aged living in the community.

Much of the actual hands-on care will ultimately be provided by family members, aides and community volunteers. Therefore, it is especially important that individuals with the appropriate knowledge and skill be available to teach those who actually provide the services to the elderly individual. When someone needs assistance getting out of bed and into a wheelchair, they have a right to expect that they will be shown the easiest, safest and most energy efficient way to accomplish the task. Likewise when they need assistance obtaining social security survivor benefits, they have a right to expect a comparable level of help in solving their problem. There are basic principles of care shared by all providers who work with the frail disabled elderly. There are also a wide variety of specific technical skills discrete to particular disciplines. A system of community care should also have the capacity to call upon the unique knowledge and skills of other disciplines when the assessment findings indicate a need for their expertise.

At this point it is appropriate to consider the reasons that occupational therapists were selected to implement this project. The director of PGA's in-home services and his staff had identified a need to enhance in-home and senior center staff's ability to work effectively with their frail disabled elderly clients. Occupational therapists' clinical skills were well suited to this need. In evaluating an individual, the occupational therapist determines:

1. the individual's current level of function in his environment
2. the individual's potential for maintaining and improving his function
3. the performance components (physical, cognitive, psychoso-

cial, etc.) that need strengthening in order to achieve as much independence of function as possible
4. the physical resources and the interpersonal factors in the environment that effect the individual's function.

In treating the individual the therapist:

1. guides the client in purposeful, self-directed, activity to improve performance and skills
2. adapts activity and equipment to make performance possible
3. modifies the environment to enable performance.

These skills, coupled with a comprehensive knowledge of disease processes and disabling conditions, were what therapists called upon in teaching in-home and senior center staff about the effects of specific disease processes and illnesses on the elderly. Staff used this knowledge to make more structured observations and to ask more appropriate questions during their assessment process. As a result they obtained a more accurate and realistic picture of the frail client's actual day-to-day performance, functional problems and service needs.

Therapists' knowledge of community resources in specific areas of health care, particularly in rehabilitation and mental health were also useful to the project. Therapists worked closely with the nurse consultants to expand the bank of information on health facilities and services available to in-home and center staffs.

While the occupational therapists were able to expand staff's understanding of the impact of specific health problems on the elderly's ability to function safely and satisfactorily in the community, they were not able to meet the elderly client's needs for specific occupational therapy services. As the project progressed, service managers, center staff and nurse consultants referred an increasing number of clients to the occupational therapists for treatment of specific disabilities and management of particular environmental problems. Project therapists estimated that they were able to handle only about 15 percent of the needs they identified among the frail disabled elderly. The project's time limited design did not permit provision of a greater amount of direct service.

This project demonstrates the effectiveness of an interdisciplinary team and points up the need for a broadly constituted interdisciplinary group of providers to staff community networks serving the frail disabled elderly. The elderly are a heterogeneous group with very diverse life styles. The frail disabled elderly are a microcosm of this larger group, reflecting a similar diversity of life style and, in addition, manifesting a diversity of need for supportive services. Provision of these services involves a whole range of social, economic and ethical issues that service providers in general, and health care providers in particular, have just begun to study. The need is evident. Service providers must act collaboratively to address these issues, to solve these problems and to provide for these needs. It is especially important to bridge the gap in knowledge and understanding that often exists among service providers from different disciplines if we are to provide humane cost effective and efficient health care to the frail disabled elderly.

REFERENCES

1. Levine, Ghita, *Long Term Care: In Search of Solutions*. National Conference on Social Welfare, 1730 M Street, N.W., Washington, D.C., 1981.
2. Butler, Robert N., *Why Survive, Being Old in America*. New York: Harper and Row, 1975.
3. Maddox, George L., "The Continuum of Care: Movement Toward the Community," in *Handbook of Geriatric Psychiatry*, eds. Edward W. Busse and Dan G. Blazer. New York: Van Nostrand Reinhold, 1980.
4. Ellis, Nancy B. and Martell, Alan, "Rotating Specialist Project in Occupational Therapy, Summary Report." The Philadelphia Corporation for Aging, 1317 Filbert Street, Philadelphia, PA. 1981.

The Continuum of Care Within Psychogeriatric Day Programming: A Study of Program Evolution

Eleanor R. Frenkel, MS
Susan R. Sherman, PhD
Evelyn S. Newman, MLS
Anthony Derico, MSW

ABSTRACT. Day programs represent an increasingly important component in treatment for the elderly. Several attempts have been made to categorize the wide variety of such programs but little attempt has been made to analyze the dynamic rather than static nature of such program design. Dalton's model of induced change is tested and illustrated through application to a psychogeriatric day program. Some of the reasons for the evolution which took place in the program included realization of the increased need to serve long-term chronic psychiatric clients, staffing changes, heterogeneity of clientele, change in availability of alternate resources in the community. The advantages of program flexibility in a developing area such as day care are discussed.

It has been stated that no continuum of long-term care services is complete without day care programming. Such programs are uniquely suited to provide and coordinate a broad range of services (Pfeiffer, 1976) and to prevent the decline of the frail elderly (Kaplan, 1976). Other benefits of day care include socialization, re-so-

---

The research was supported by the NRTA/AARP Andrus Foundation. The authors wish to acknowledge the assistance of Erica Sufrin, Sarah Traynor and the staff of the Geriatric Unit. An earlier version of this paper was presented at Symposium on Geriatric Day Care: Definitional Issues, at the Northeastern Gerontological Society, April 29, 1982, Albany, New York.

Eleanor R. Frenkel, Coordinator of Elderly Services, Jewish Community Council of Washington Heights-Inwood, 121 Bennett Avenue, New York, NY 10033. Susan R. Sherman, Associate Professor, School of Social Welfare, Evelyn S. Newman, Research Associate, Ringel Institute of Gerontology, at SUNY/Albany, 135 Western Avenue, Albany, NY 12222. Anthony Derico is a Psychiatric Social Worker, Capital District Psychiatric Center, Albany, NY.

17

cialization, life satisfaction (Rathbone-McCuan, 1973), increased self-esteem (Kaplan, 1976) and improvement in quality of life (Connecticut Department of Aging, 1979). Further, day programs provide respite to families caring for disabled elderly and may thus delay the need for institutionalization.

Day programs, however, differ greatly in both the kinds of services provided and types of clients served. Much of the literature distinguishes two models of programs (Padula, 1972; Pickett, 1979; Rathbone-McCuan, 1973; Weissert, 1976). The models have been variously called Model I: Day Hospital; and Model II: Day Care, Multipurpose or Maintenance Centers. These models differentiate primarily between therapeutic environments and those which provide for social support and activities. It is of note that not all programs fall clearly into either one of these distinct categories and some, such as psychiatric day programs, are omitted from either model.

Other classifications of programs do exist. The Department of Health and Human Services (1980), in its Directory of Adult Day Centers classified programs into three types: restorative, maintenance and social. Weiler and Rathbone-McCuan (1978), in recognition of the degree of flexibility of day programs and the extent of overlap between models have classified four service modalities: day hospital; social/health center; psycho-social center; and social center.

In actuality, programs vary greatly as to the types of services they provide (Pickett, 1979; Weiler & Rathbone-McCuan, 1978; Weissert, 1976). Although day care overall offers this great degree of diversity, individual programs tend to follow one model and may offer a more limited range of services. This restriction to one model has, however, been considered unrealistic (Trager, 1976), as combinations of program models providing a continuum of care can greatly broaden the services provided in a particular community.

Complementary social day centers, for example, are described as essential to the proper functioning of a day hospital by Brocklehurst (1970) and Robins (1975). Lorenze, Hamill, and Oliver (1974) emphasize the importance of free movement to the appropriate level of care within day care centers for discharged day hospital patients.

It is, however, often difficult to operationalize and implement theoretical program models of service delivery. In fact, much has been written regarding what has been called the "slippage between intent and action" in the development of social programs (Weiss,

1972, p. 97)). Blumer (1971), for example, notes that as a new program plan is put into effect it is ". . . modified, twisted and reshaped, and takes on unforeseen accretions" (p. 304). There is a paucity of literature describing the development and implementation of day programs. Particularly lacking is systematic information describing program implementation within the context of a theoretical model. One theoretical model which may help formulate a description of such development is proposed by Dalton (1970). Dalton describes the process of organizational change and development in light of a theoretical model of induced change which involves four steps: (1) tension in the system; (2) intervention of a prestigious influencing agent; (3) individuals' attempts to implement the proposed changes; and (4) new behavior and attitudes. As policy dictates the implementation of new programs it is important to understand the pressures which cause them finally to assume the shape they do. This paper examines some of the intervening factors which underlay the modifications of one such program. The information reported is based on a larger study of psychogeriatric day care at a state psychiatric center. Elsewhere we have described the influence of one aspect of a program, staff classification decisions, on the course of the implementation of a continuum of care day program (Frenkel et al., in press). The present paper further describes the implementation of that program with special emphasis on its evolution through unexpected pressures and demands.

THE SETTING

The study was conducted at the Geriatric Unit of a State Psychiatric Center. At the outset of the study a number of levels of care were available.

1. *Day Hospital (DH):* a treatment oriented psychiatric day program for psychiatrically impaired non-institutionalized elderly persons. Attendance varied from 1/2 to 3 1/2 days per week.
2. *Geriatric Day Care (DC)*: a program of structured activities including group discussions of common problems or current events, recreational and activity therapies, trips, and training in self-maintenance activities of daily living should the need arise. Attendance varied from 1/2 to 3 1/2 days per week.
3. *Community Management*: residence within the community

with the provision of consultation services by the staff of the Geriatric Unit. This involves, as needed, prescription of psychotropic and other medications, supportive follow-up and periodic reassessment. Persons in this group have access to the day programs and all services of the Unit.

4. *Inpatient Unit*: Day program clients may be moved to Inpatient Units within the facility as the need for additional support or supervision arises, and inpatients may attend the day program.

5. *Potpourri Program*: an age-integrated non-structured activities program which serves the entire psychiatric center. Geriatric Unit clients may attend Potpourri concurrently with their geriatric day programs or they may be discharged into this program. Potpourri serves as a sheltered environment which eases the transition into the community.

Clients may remain in any of these treatment modes for as long as necessary, and they may be transferred back and forth as the need arises.

At the beginning of the study the Geriatric Unit's professional staff consisted of three social workers, three community mental health nurses, a consulting psychiatrist and a clinical psychologist who was the Unit chief.

DESCRIPTION OF THE PROGRAM'S EVOLUTION

When the study began both the DH program, which served primarily acute and some chronic psychiatric clients, and a DC program which served primarily clients with mild to moderate organic brain syndrome (OBS) were in place in the Geriatric Unit. The two programs could best be described in terms of a horizontal arrangement of levels of care; the programs complemented each other by serving client populations whose needs differed sufficiently to require different services. In this scheme there is no expectation that clients move from one program to another as neither program serves people who are more or less impaired but rather people who have different patterns of impairment. Such a scheme does not preclude movement between programs; movement may occur as the client's condition changes but this would constitute an exceptional case rather than an expected outcome of treatment.

As time went on the psychiatric center administration saw a need to focus attention on the long-term, chronic psychiatric clients. These clients were similar to the OBS clients already in day care in that both were seen as not requiring active psychotherapy and both could benefit from structured activities and socialization programs. There are, however, differences in the types of specific activities which could be most beneficial to each group. For example, reality orientation was seen as appropriate for OBS clients and not necessary for the chronic psychiatric patients.

Thus, in order to serve the chronic psychiatric patients, many of whom were already in the DH, a new day care program (which had existed several years before but had been discontinued) was reinstituted to replace the DC which was already in existence. It was expected that the new program would be less custodial and would provide clients with activities, socialization, and a supportive environment and thus prevent future institutionalization. The program could also serve as a transition to the community for those who had previously been institutionalized.

This DC program was expected to relate to the DH in what could be represented as a vertical arrangement of levels of care: the programs complement each other by providing more or less intensive care for the same or similar clients as their needs change. This scheme is similar to the arrangements described in Brocklehurst (1970) and Robins (1975), where day centers serve as transitions from the therapeutic environment of day hospitals into the community.

The course of events described thus far corresponds to the first two stages of Dalton's model of induced change. First, tension was experienced in the system by the realization of the need to serve the long-term chronic psychiatric clients. Secondly, the psychiatric center administration intervened and encouraged the development of a new program (or in this case the restructuring of an existing program) to resolve the tension. As will be described later, this move created its own tensions.

To implement the program, staff and scheduling changes were made. A number of OBS clients were moved to other settings and the remainder were included in the new DC program as it was felt that its activities were not overly demanding and the program could accommodate to their needs as well.

Shortly after the implementation of the new program, new tensions arose which redirected the course of its development. The first of the tensions is the heterogeneity of the clientele, coupled with insufficient staff to allow for meeting diverse needs of DC participants.

From its inception, the new DC program served a diverse population. Fifty-three percent were borderline or OBS (as measured by Kahn et al., 1960) while 43% had previous psychiatric hospitalization. The DC clients were least able to perform ADL independently, with the staff reporting only 24% as completely independent. The heterogeneity of the DC program's clientele and insufficient staff presented a number of difficulties for its implementation. Although both the OBS and the chronic psychiatric clients required socialization and structured activities, impairments in ADL skills and confusion on the part of OBS clients limited the types of activities which could be conducted. For example, resocialization activities such as shopping or restaurant outings were considered very valuable to the chronic psychiatric clients but inappropriate for the OBS clients who needed intensive supervision at all times. Thus, on some days the group was divided so that, for example, the less organically impaired clients could go on trips while the others remained behind. However, there were not enough staff members to conduct two separate programs and the program gradually was restructured to meet the needs of the most organically impaired group, rather than the chronic psychiatric clients.

In addition, a number of other tensions contributed to the change in the program. A major factor was the types of available resources within the community. As described above, when the DC program began, it was decided that it was to focus on the chronic psychiatric population though those with mild OBS would not be completely excluded. During the time of the program's development, however, there were no resources to deal with the OBS client living within the community and thus, the Geriatric Unit constantly received referrals of OBS clients needing treatment. The referrals came both from the outside community and from other units within the psychiatric center.

The number of OBS clients in the program further increased because a number of people already in a program, either in DH or DC, also developed impairments typical of OBS in addition to their psychiatric problems. A similar situation arose with regard to people referred for admission; their primary problem may have been psychiatric, making them appropriate for the Geriatric Unit program, but they also had secondary problems relating to OBS. As there were no other community resources to serve this group, the Geriatric Unit was under increasing pressure to include them in the DC program.

Not only did the lack of alternative services for OBS clients affect the composition of the program, but the availability of such alternative programs for the chronic psychiatric clients had a similar effect. An important resource was the geriatric hostel which opened shortly after the inception of the new DC program. This hostel is a supervised community residence where the residents share in the tasks of daily living, and receive individual and group counseling and support by staff members and support agencies. Fourteen Geriatric Unit clients were moved into this hostel at the time of its opening—most of these came from the DC program.

Another alternative service available to chronic psychiatric clients is the age-integrated Potpourri Program described above. This program was especially well suited for those clients who had moved to the geriatric hostel. These clients also had access to CM which involves prescription of medications, supportive follow-up and periodic reassessment. According to program staff, the combination of the supervision of the hostel, activities of Potpourri and access to CM was optimal for this group. The Potpourri Club allowed for a greater degree of independence than did the structured DC program and most clients adapted well to the expectations and demands of their new situation. Clients who resisted moving out of the program or who needed additional support were given the option of attending DH.

A third source of tension in addition to client heterogeneity and the distribution of local resources which served to restructure the program was staff attitudes. The diverse professional staff brought to their professional judgments the perspectives of their disciplines and past experiences. There were, in fact, conflicting opinions among the clinicians regarding the nature of the DC program and the types of clients who could best be served by the program. One group felt that the program should only serve psychiatrically impaired clients. Other clinicians were particularly concerned about serving OBS clients who could not receive help elsewhere in the community. These clinicians actively advocated for the inclusion of OBS clients in the program. As the Unit Guidelines allowed for the inclusion of clients with mild to moderate OBS and since many were referred to the Unit, the number of these clients in the program constantly increased.

As a result of differences in staff opinions regarding program emphasis and of the continuing pressure of community demands, criteria for determining placement were never clearly defined. In the absence of clear criteria, clinicians used different and often inconsistent classification criteria in assigning clients to programs. For example, history of psychiatric treatment was judged by clinicians to be one of the least relevant factors in their classification decisions, despite the fact that the chronic/acute psychiatric distinction was intended as an essential difference between DH and DC clients (Frenkel et al., in press).

It must be emphasized that none of the tensions discussed above occurred in isolation; rather each was part of a "snowball effect." As more OBS clients entered the program a smaller percentage of the clients were able to participate in planned activities such as discussion groups. Accommodations had to be made to meet the needs of the OBS clients; for example, reality orientation was introduced. As a result of this gradual shift in the nature of the program, those people for whom DC was originally designed (i.e., chronic psychiatric patients) became less suited for the program as it actually existed. This provided an incentive for staff to move such clients to more appropriate settings. When DC became increasingly appropriate for OBS persons, resistance to admission of such clients declined, and their numbers within the program rose further. It was apparent that the absence of clear-cut classification criteria allowed for the inclusion of OBS clients, and the presence of these clients further encouraged flexibility in admissions to allow for the inclusion of additional OBS clients.

Thus, after a year and a half the program at the Geriatric Unit had almost come full circle. The DH served functionally disabled psychiatric clients; the DC program served clients with mild to moderate organic brain syndrome. The CM program in conjunction with the Potpourri Club and the Geriatric Hostel, served chronic psychiatric clients whose primary need was for socialization and activity. Shifting these chronic patients from DH to DC and finally to the less structured program is expected to facilitate the future movement of these chronic psychiatric clients to community groups such as senior centers. With this latest move the Geriatraic Unit is once again in a position to provide a DC program for frail elderly with some level of organic brain syndrome, a group which is not presently served by other community resources. The services at the Unit had evolved from an original horizontal to a vertical and back to a horizontal continuum of care. It appears that an equilibrium was reached once again.

The overall change which had occurred at the Geriatric Unit represents a departure from Dalton's model of change in that it was not a directed or induced change but rather a gradual evolution in response to internal and external tensions. The evolution occurred without the intervention of a particular influencing agent, although a number of clinicians contributed indirectly through their admissions and classification decisions.

Worthy of note, too, is the interplay between the clinicians, the Unit Chief and the top administration of the Psychiatric Center. During the period in which the day program was evolving, the Unit Chief left and was replaced. Staff changes were also occurring throughout the facility administration. It is not known how much of the return to the original design can be attributed to the personal philosophy of the new staff and the way they perceived the needs of the community, or whether it was simply easier to accede to the practices of staff and their definitions of criteria and programming given the state of flux.

Discussion

The course of the evolution of the Geriatric Unit program is not unique. Program changes occur which are not always intended and by the same token, planned changes often do not take place. The evolution described here can be viewed from two opposite perspectives. The first perspective views this evolution from a managerial perspective as an expression of inability to implement a program change. In terms of Dalton's model, the process of change was arrested at Stage 3; attempts were made to implement the proposed change but they never resulted in Stage 4, the acquisition of new behaviors and attitudes. A possible explanation for such a failure would be resistance on the part of some clinicians who did not perceive the need for the program change.

Further, while the planned change might have been accomplished more successfully through the early development of clear-cut criteria for admission into each program as stated above, staff members differed in their perceptions of goals and of clients to be served by the program. As the criteria for admission into the program were very broad, clients with varied needs were grouped together. Definite program goals and criteria for admission are essential especially when resources and staff are limited.

In the field of day care, however, where models for programs are just now emerging, there is a great need to serve a wide range of clients, and too rigid program definitions may be premature and constraining. Program adaptability and flexibility are essential in such an emerging field. In fact, such flexibility has been described as a major strength of day care programs (Trager, 1976).

The evolution of the Geriatric Unit's program can also be viewed from a programmatic perspective recognizing the flexibility of day care. From this perspective, the evolution represents the successful fulfillment of the potential for adaptability. The program gradually changed to adjust to the needs of both its current clients and those in the community who could benefit from participation. The basic components of a day care program were available and could be used by both types of clients: the chronic psychiatric patients or OBS clients. It was only particular activities such as reality orientation or discussion groups which required change. This was accomplished with minimum disruption.

This paper has described the development and implementation of a continuum of care day care program in terms of a theoretical model of organizational change. The course of development of the program, however, did not correspond completely to the theoretical model. It is hoped that the paper has served to highlight the dynamic nature of a program such as day care and to raise questions regarding tensions which affect implementation.

REFERENCES

Blumer, H. Social problems as collective behavior. *Social Problems*, 1971, *18*, 298-306.
Brocklehurst, J.C. *The geriatric day hospital.* London: King Edwards Hospital Fund, 1970.
Dalton, G.W. Influence and organizational change. In G.W. Dalton and P.R. Lawrence (Eds.), *Organizational change and development.* Homewood, Illinois: Richard D. Irwin, 1970.
Department of Health and Human Services, Health Standards and Quality Bureau, *Directory of adult day centers.* Baltimore, Maryland, 1980.
Frenkel, E.R., Newman, E.S., & Sherman, S.R. Classification decisions within psychogeriatric day care, in press.
Kahn, R.L., Goldfarb, A.I., Pollack, M., & Peck, A. Brief objective measures for the determination of mental status in the aged. *American Journal of Psychiatry*, 1960, *117*, 326-328.
Kaplan, J. Goals of day care: Restoration of function and maintenance and prevention of decline. In E. Pfeiffer (Ed.), *Daycare for older adults: A conference report.* Center for the Study of Aging and Human Development, Duke University, 1976.

Lorenze, E.J., Hamill, C.M., & Oliver, R.C. The day hospital: An alternative to institutional care. *Journal of American Geriatrics Society*, 1974, *22*, 316-319.

Padula, H. Developing day care for older people. *Technical Assistance Monograph*, NCOA, September, 1972.

Pfeiffer, E. Range and scope of daycare services. In E. Pfeiffer (Ed), *Daycare for older adults: A conference report*. Center for the Study of Aging and Human Development, Duke University, 1976.

Pickett, M. Day treatment for the elderly: An overview. Institute of Gerontology, School of Social Welfare, State University of New York at Albany, 1979.

Rathbone-McCuan, E. An evaluation of a geriatric day care center as a parallel service to institutional care. Project of the Levindale Geriatric Research Center, Baltimore, Maryland, 1973.

Robins, E.G. Report on day hospitals in Israel and Great Britain. Division of Long Term Care, National Center for Health Services Research, HRA, DHEW, 1975.

State of Connecticut, Department of Aging. Adult day care in Connecticut. Report to the General Assembly, September 1979.

Trager, B. Adult day care facilities for treatment, health care and related services, a working paper. Prepared for Special Committee on Aging—U.S. Senate, September 1976.

Weiler, P.G., & Rathbone-McCuan, E. *Adult day care: community work with the elderly*. New York: Springer, 1978.

Weiss, C.H. *Evaluation research: Methods for assessing program effectiveness*. New Jersey: Prentice-Hall, 1972.

Weissert, G. A final report—Adult day care in the United States: A comparative study. National Center for Health Services Research, HRA-Department of Health, Education and Welfare, 1976.

A Comparison of the Effectiveness of Various Approaches to Visiting Isolated Community Elderly

Robert J. Calsyn, PhD
Michelle Munson
David Peaco
Janet Kupferberg
Jean Jackson

ABSTRACT. Two studies were conducted evaluating the effectiveness of friendly visitor programs in increasing clients' life satisfaction. Study 1 found no difference between face-to-face visiting, phone visiting, and a no treatment control on client life satisfaction. Study 2 found a marginally significant difference in favor of a personal history approach over a companionship approach to visiting in increasing client life satisfaction. Clients' living situation (alone or with others) had no effect on changes in life satisfaction in Study 1. However, in Study 2 clients who lived with someone increased their life satisfaction more than clients who lived alone.

The negative consequences of social isolation of the elderly has been a focus in gerontological research for at least thirty years. The work of Bennett (1980) and her colleagues as well as that of Lowenthal and Boler (1965) and Lowenthal and Havens (1968) has consistently shown that social isolation due to losses such as death of a spouse, retirement, and failing health is correlated with a decline in morale and/or psychological adjustment. Similarly research on the correlates of life satisfaction in the elderly has consistently found a modest correlation between social activity and life satisfaction (Larson, 1978).

Reprint requests should be sent to Dr. Calsyn, Psychology Department, University of Missouri-St. Louis, 8001 Natural Bridge Road, St. Louis, MO 63121.

We would like to thank Mrs. Valerie Wooten and Jeanette Collins for typing this manuscript, and Kathy Corbett for serving as the history consultant to the project.

Many communities have developed "friendly visitor" programs staffed by volunteers or paraprofessionals who visit the isolated elderly on a regular basis in an attempt to improve the morale of the elderly. Despite their popularity we are aware of only three studies which have evaluated the effectiveness of "friendly visitor" programs. Two of the studies were done in nursing homes and one study was done with elderly living in the community. Both studies (Arthur, Donnan, & Lair, 1973; Reinke, Holmes, & Denney, 1981) with nursing home patients found that patients who received visitors had better morale than control group patients without visitors. The evaluators (Mulligan & Bennett, 1977) of the friendly visitor program for community based elderly concluded that their program had a positive impact on the mental status, grooming, and apartment upkeep of visited clients compared to non-visited controls. Unfortunately, several methodological problems render their results questionable including preprogram differences between treatment and control clients, inappropriate statistical analyses, and the fact that the visitors themselves rated both treatment and control clients on the outcome measures. Clearly, more studies are needed to evaluate the effectiveness of "friendly visitor" programs, particularly with elderly living in the community.

Although the scope of services provided by telephone reassurance programs for the elderly varies from community to community, many programs have reducing social isolation as one of their goals and encourage callers to "visit" on the phone with their clients. Since telephone programs are less expensive and can potentially reach more clients because travel time is eliminated and visitors without transportation can be utilized, comparing the relative effectiveness of face-to-face visiting and phone visiting has important practical significance. Study 1 compares face-to-face visiting against phone visiting and a no treatment control group in a true experiment.

Most "friendly visitor" programs including those that were reviewed above employ a present-oriented companionship approach to visiting. Visitors are encouraged to focus on current concerns of their clients, engage them in conversation about current events, and involve them in games or crafts. In contrast to this present-oriented approach are techniques which encourage clients to reminisce about the past (Lewis & Butter, 1974; Pincus, 1970). These approaches regard the tendency of older persons to reminisce as a natural process that should be nurtured and facilitated rather than discouraged.

Paging through scrapbooks and old photo albums, tracing one's geneology, and dictating one's family history, are seen as potential therapeutic tools. To the authors' knowledge no empirical research has been conducted on the relative efficacy of these life review or reminiscing techniques in working with the elderly. Certainly no comparative research has been done comparing a companionship approach which emphasizes the present with a more past oriented, reminiscing type of treatment program. Study 2 compared a fairly standard companionship type of "friendly visitor" program against a personal history approach to visiting.

Although our initial plan was to serve only the elderly who lived alone, our referral sources contended that they had many elderly clients who lived with others who were just as isolated as elderly live-alones. In many of these cases economic or health problems had necessitated the elderly client moving in with the family of one of their children. Lowenthal and Boler's (1965) finding that 40% of the involuntarily isolated lived with others as compared to 19% of the voluntarily isolated and 29% of the non-isolated supported the contention of our referral sources that living with others does not guarantee non-isolation. Although we agreed to accept clients who lived with others, we were apprehensive about the ability of our visitors to intervene in family situations where considerable domestic strain might exist. We felt that our various treatments would be more effective with clients who lived alone. Thus, we predicted a treatment by living situation interaction in Study 1 and a main effect of living situation in Study 2.

METHOD

Study 1

Participants. Clients were referred by a number of agencies serving the elderly, including the Meals on Wheels Program and the County Older Residents Program. All of the clients lived in noninstitutional settings. Some of the clients lived alone; others lived with their family or a roommate. All of the clients were considered socially isolated by the referral source. Sometimes the isolation was due to physical mobility problems; other times fear of crime, loss of a significant other, strain in the family, or other reasons led the referral source to describe the potential client as socially isolated. After referral clients were interviewed by one of the junior authors who obtained informed consent, learned client's preferences regarding type of visitor, and administered the pretest. A total of 58 people (47 females and 11 males) agreed to participate in the program. However, eight people did not provide posttest data; four of these people in the phone condition dropped out of the program after only a few visits; and the remaining four people did not complete the posttest due to death or illness. The average age of the participants was 76.77.

Design. A 3x2 analysis of covariance design was employed in Study 1. The two factors were treatment condition (face-to-face visiting, phone visiting, and no treatment control) and living situation (alone or with someone). Participants in the no treatment control condition received a face-to-face visitor at the conclusion of the study. The dependent variable was life-satisfaction as measured by the LSIZ (Wood, Wylie, & Sheafer, 1966). Respondents respond agree, uncertain or disagree to thirteen statements such as "This is the dreariest time of my life," and "I've gotten pretty much what I expected out of life." Items are scored in such a way that higher total scores indicate more life satisfaction. The pretest score on the LSIZ was the covariate. Cronbach alpha for the LSIZ was .57 at both the pretest and the posttest for the combined samples used in Study 1 and Study 2. Pretesting occurred approximately two weeks before the first visit and posttesting about two weeks after the last visit. In order to randomly assign clients to treatment conditions and at the same time honor client preferences with regard to race and/or sex of the visitor as well as visitor preferences with regard to geographic area they were willing to visit, it was necessary to put clients in blocks prior to random assignment. For example, there were blocks of clients who requested a white visitor and blocks of clients who requested a female visitor, and blocks of clients by geographic area. Then visitors were assigned to a given block based on the visitor's sex and/or race and the visitor's geographic preference. Within blocks clients were then randomly assigned to one of the treatment conditions. There were 16 blocks of three clients that were randomly assigned to one of the three treatment conditions. These were five blocks of only two clients; clients in these blocks were randomly assigned to either face-to-face visiting or phone visiting. This was done in order to maximize the number of clients who could be visited by our 21 visitors and still maintain random assignment.

Visitor recruitment and training. Older volunteers referred by senior citizen organizations and undergraduate students enrolled in a field placement course served as visitors in this study. There were 14 female and 7 male visitors. All potential visitors were interviewed by one of the authors regarding their interest in the program, prior experience, and career aspirations. At this point, four potential visitors chose not to continue in the project. Training consisted of three four-hour sessions. Both didactic and experiential exercises were included. During the first session, information on the biological, psychological, and social aspects of aging was presented. Emphasis was placed on the number of losses that confront the elderly and the accompanying grief reaction to those losses. Visitors were then given the opportunity to express their own feelings about aging and death and to share with the group their experiences with the elderly. Time was also devoted to establishing the ground rules for the visiting in terms of keeping appointments, types of activities that were permissible, and potential legal issues such as liability in case of an accident. The second and third training sessions were devoted to learning and practicing communication skills. The active listening approach of Gordon (1970) was the primary communication technique taught. Emphasis was placed on listening for feelings and reflecting those feelings back to the client. Visitors were discouraged from giving advice prematurely and urged to let decision-making remain in the client's control. Role playing was used extensively; volunteers took turns playing both the client role and the helper role. Feedback was provided by both trainers and other group members.

Visits and supervision. Clients were visited once a week for a period of twelve weeks. The length of visit varied from client to client and from week to week, but generally face-to-face visits lasted about 1½ hours per visit and phone visits lasted about 45 minutes. Each visitor had one face-to-face client and one phone client. Visitors engaged in a variety of activities with their clients including helping with activities of daily living such as shopping as well as some advocacy work with agencies such as the Social Security Administration and public aid. However, most of the visiting time was spent in companionship activities, primarily talking about common interests.

Visitors were required to turn in a journal sheet on each of their visits. These sheets contained information regarding activities that occurred during the visits, information on any new problems that the client might be facing, as well as the volunteer's feelings about the visit. These journal sheets were turned in at bi-weekly supervision sessions. These supervision sessions were small group sessions of six to eight members led by one of the authors. Each client was discussed at each meeting. Group members tried to give each other support and suggestions on more effective ways of communication, as well as suggestions regarding activities to do on the visit and/or agencies which might provide needed services. The last two sessions focused on termination issues.

Study 2

Participants and design. Clients were referred by the same agencies as in Study 1. All lived in noninstitutional settings and were considered socially isolated by the referral source. Informed consent and administration of the pretest was conducted in the same manner as in Study 1. A total of 34 people (28 females and 6 males) agreed to participate in the study. The average age of participants was 77.34 years. None of these people had participated in Study 1, and all clients were visited on a face-to-face basis. A 2x2 analysis of covariance design was used. The two factors were treatment condition (companionship approach or personal history approach) and living condition (alone or with someone). Life satisfaction as measured by the LSIZ was the dependent variable and the covariate was the pretest assessment on the LSIZ. The pretest occurred approximately two weeks before the first visit and the posttest occurred approximately two weeks after the last visit. As in Study 1 clients were put in blocks prior to random assignment in order to honor client and visitor preferences. There were two clients per block. After visitors had been assigned to a block consistent with client and visitor preferences, the two clients within each block were randomly assigned to one of the two treatment conditions. The blocking variable was not included as a factor in the analysis. One client in the companionship condition could not be posttested due to illness.

Visitor recruitment and training. Undergraduate students (11 females and 6 males) enrolled in a field placement course served as visitors in the study. Screening of visitors was done in the same manner as Study 1. As in Study 1 training consisted of three four hour sessions. Sessions 1 and 2 were identical to sessions 1 and 2 in Study 1. However, rather than receiving additional practice in active listening, session three was devoted to training in personal history techniques. The session was led by a research associate from the history department who had considerable experience in various oral history projects including one with retired members of the Ladies Garment Workers Union. Topics covered in the training included kinds of materials that can be used in assembling a personal history (e.g., family photographs, family documents, newspaper clippings, memorabilia, as well as structured interviews). Some time was also devoted to discussion of general topics that might be relevant to a large segment of the client population (e.g., the depression of the 1930s, World Wars I and II, living on a farm, labor union experiences and the St. Louis World's Fair). Specific information on tape-recording and transcribing tapes was also discussed and written handouts passed out. Considerable emphasis was placed on structured interviewing techniques with particular emphasis on sequencing of questions, use of the open ended question, the use of probes, and helping the client integrate the experience. Several students then took turns interviewing the trainer regarding her experiences as a child during World War II.

Visits and supervision. Clients were visited once a week for a period of twelve weeks. The length of visits varied from client to client and from week to week but averaged 1½ hours per visit. Each visitor had one client in each of the two conditions. In the companionship condition visitors engaged in activities similar to those described in Study 1. In the personal history condition visitors were required to develop a personal history project with their client. Visitors were requested to make at least three tape recordings to this end and had to produce a written product consisting in part of an edited transcription of the tapes which they gave their personal history client at the end of the twelve weeks.

As in Study 1 visitors were required to turn in a journal sheet on each of their visits and to attend bi-weekly supervision sessions. In addition, the history consultant provided individual supervision as needed with regard to selecting interview topics, development of the interview protocol, and transcribing tapes for the personal history client.

RESULTS

Study 1. Table 1 contains the pretest and posttest group means on the life satisfaction measures for Study 1 participants. The analysis of covariance indicated no significant treatment effect ($F = .34$,

Table 1

Study 1 pretest and posttest means and standard deviations on the life satisfaction measure.

	Living Situation			
	Alone		With Someone	
Condition	Pre	Post	Pre	Post
Companion				
Mean	13.55	14.36	11.70	10.70
S.D.	3.45	3.41	3.59	5.95
N		11		10
Phone				
Mean	13.00	13.22	15.14	15.14
S.D.	4.97	2.91	3.72	3.28
N		9		7
Control				
Mean	13.63	14.50	12.20	12.80
S.D.	3.96	3.16	4.21	2.95
N		8		5

$p < .71$), no significant effect of living condition ($F = 1.47$, $p < .23$), and no significant interaction ($F = 1.13$, $p < .33$). While, there were no significant differences between face-to-face visiting and phone visiting on the life satisfaction measure, it is important to note the clients and visitors alike expressed considerable frustration with the phone visits. As noted earlier four clients in the phone condition dropped out of the project.

Study 2. Table 2 displays the pretest and posttest group means on the life satisfaction for Study 2 participants. The analysis of covariance indicated a marginally significant treatment effect ($F =$

3.13, $p < .08$), such that clients in the personal history condition increased their life satisfaction more than clients in the companionship condition. There was a significant effect of living condition ($F = 5.07$, $p < .03$), such that clients who lived with someone increased their life satisfaction more than clients who lived alone. There was no significant interaction ($F = .01$, $p < .91$).

DISCUSSION

Although companionship oriented friendly visitor programs appear to be effective in increasing the morale of institutionalized elderly (Arthur, Donnan, & Lair, 1973; Reinke, Holmes, & Denney, 1981) our two studies found companionship oriented friendly visiting to having no effect on the life satisfaction of noninstitutionalized elderly. Thus, to date only one study (Mulligan & Bennett, 1977) has reported positive effects of a companionship oriented friendly visitor program on the noninstitutionalized elderly and that study is

Table 2

Study 2 pretest and posttest means and standard deviations on the life satisfaction measure.

	Living Situation			
	Alone		With Someone	
Condition	Pre	Post	Pre	Post
Companion				
Mean	12.87	12.62	16.75	18.13
S.D.	6.62	4.69	3.88	4.22
N	8		8	
History				
Mean	14.64	16.18	14.83	18.60
S.D.	7.50	5.56	4.22	6.19
N	11		6	

too flawed methodologically to put much confidence in its conclusions.

The fact that the personal history treatment had a marginally significant effect on the life satisfaction of the elderly is an encouraging finding. One explanation for the superiority of the personal history approach in improving life satisfaction is that this technique allows the client to review his/her past and achieve some sort of integrated resolution. In addition, the tape recordings and written document provided concrete evidence that the personal history visits accomplished something worthwhile. Some visitors and clients in the companionship condition exchanged pictures or inexpensive gifts so as to have a permanent reminder that the experience had been worthwhile.

It is also our opinion that the relationship between visitor and client was more reciprocal in the personal history condition than the companionship condition. Rather than always receiving help clients in the personal history condition were helping the visitor with a school project and educating the visitor about some aspect of the past. Although we have no supporting empirical data, it is our opinion that clients in both conditions had more positive outcomes the more reciprocal the relationship was between client and visitor. Even our very poorest clients were happier if they could do something for the visitor or give some token of appreciation such as a homemade pie. Some of our visitors were quite adept at finding ways to make the relationship more reciprocal and change the relationship from client/helper to mutual friends. For example, one visitor who had poor writing skills used her retired teacher client to help revise her class assignments.

Although the personal history treatment appears to have some positive effect on life satisfaction, the effect is not large probably due to the fact the intervention only ends the client's social isolation for 1½ hours per week. It could be argued that friendly visitors might better spend their time trying to find ways for the client to increase their social interactions throughout the remainder of the week. Some researchers (Harris & Bodden, 1978; Rosen & Rosen, 1982; Weiner, 1980) have provided evidence that structured group experiences with other elderly clients have increased the morale of noninstitutionalized elderly. Our visitors did try to get their clients to attend senior citizen centers, and other social groups, often offering to accompany their clients to the initial group meetings. Most of our clients rejected the suggestion to attend group functions, citing either lack of interest in the activities of the group or concerns about their own appearance, physical ability, and/or mental capabilities.

Our results are equivocal with respect to the effect of living situation (alone or with others) on life satisfaction. In Study 1 there was no main effect of living situation or treatment by living situation interaction. However, in Study 2 contrary to our prediction clients who lived with someone increased their life satisfaction significantly more than clients who lived alone. Contrary to our worst fears the people living with our clients welcomed the visitors. Although clients and family members frequently complained about each other in front of the visitor, the visits provided a temporary respite from the domestic strain that existed. Perhaps one of the reasons that we did not find consistent effects of living situation on life satisfaction across studies is that many of the client's who lived alone also were involved in negative interactions with their families. Many of our clients were angry at their children for not visiting them often enough; similarly, children of our clients often treated their parents as incompetents, often scolding them, and making decisions about their parents' living conditions without consultation.

Future research. Our results suggest several directions for future research. We have argued that one possible reason for the success of the personal history over the companionship approach is that it promotes a more reciprocal relationship between client and visitor. Future research employing content analyses of tapes and/or self-reports of clients and visitors could determine the level of reciprocity in the relationship and then correlate the reciprocity score with changes in clients' morale. The relationship of other dimensions of social support to changes in morale could also be examined (Mitchell & Trickett, 1980). For example, is emotional support more important than cognitive guidance or tasks assistance? Similarly, are relationships that are multidimensional more helpful than undimensional relationships? The new measures of social support that have been developed recently (Barrera, 1981) could also be used to measure how the friendly visiting experience alters the other relationships in the clients' lives.

Although in our program we attempt to match clients and visitors on the basis of expressed interest and other preferences as well as demographic characteristics of the visitors, we do not have a systematic formula for matching clients and visitors. We did do one study (Peaco, 1980) examining the effects of client/visitor matching in terms of age and sex on improving client morale.

We found no effects. Similarly, we found only marginal effects in terms of how well various volunteer personality characteristics predicted client improvement. Our only finding was that volunteers who have a low need for clarity were somehwat more effective than volunteers who needed a lot of structure. Clearly more research in this area is needed.

Treatment recommendations. Implicit in the discussion of our results is our belief that friendly visitor programs are more effective the more reciprocal client/visitor relationships are. Friendly visitors should be encouraged to search out what interests and life experiences their clients have had and then based on their own interests and needs find some areas where the client can teach or otherwise do something for the visitor. Similarly, even though many of our clients were economically disadvantaged we soon found out that it is important for the self-respect of many clients that they somehow "pay" for the service. It may be partial monetary payment (e.g., leaving the tip at a restaurant) or exchange of goods (e.g., giving the visitor a recipe). One of our clients insisted on giving the visitor surplus cheese she received. The client couldn't use the cheese because of her medication so the visitor accepted.

Similarly, it is important for visitors to allow clients to do as much for themselves as possible and not foster dependency. This frequently results in more time being consumed to complete a task (e.g., shopping) but is essential for the clients' dignity.

Termination in any helping relationship is always an important issue. Clients who have been in the program for some time have learned to anticipate the end of the semester and frequently bring up the issue of termination with their student visitors. However, we also require visitors to initiate the discussion of termination at least two weeks before the last visit. For many of the relationships termination is a misnomer, because the visitors and clients maintain some sort of contact after the conclusion of the semester. We do not discourage this, but only insist that the students not make commitments that they cannot keep. The typical form of post-course contact is phone contact and/or the student telling the client to call them for help in case of an emergency. We have found these post-course contacts to be particularly meaningful to the clients, because such contact is freely given, i.e., not required for course credit. Program directors do have to be careful about not fostering competition between the new visitor and a previous visitor. For this reason we encourage the outgoing visitor to keep contacts during the initial weeks of the new semester to a minimum. To date we have had only minor instances where a client will talk incessantly about her "wonderful" previous visitor to the new visitor. Finally, if a client/visitor relationship has become so rewarding for both parties and the student is willing to continue seeing the client on a weekly basis for no credit, we encourage them to do so and do not assign a new visitor. We use occasional phone contact with client and visitor to monitor these relationships.

Finally, our experience has reinforced the importance of regular supervision of visitors. No matter how thorough the training experience, visitors need specific guidance in forming a helping relationship that is compatible with their own personal style and the needs of the clients. We have found a bi-weekly group supervision of 5-7 visitors to be a very effective and efficient way to monitor client/visitor progress. In the initial meetings particularly it is important for the group leader to have group process goals as primary. Encourage members to share experiences with each other and seek advice from peers. If the group leader gives too much directive guidance, the session ends up being a series of one-on-one supervisions with group members being fairly passive when they are not discussing their own clients.

REFERENCES

1. Arthur, G., Donnan, H. and Lair, C. Companionship therapy with the nursing home aged. *Gerontologist*, 1973, *13*, 167-170.
2. Barrera, M. Social support in the adjustment of pregnant adolescents. In B.H. Gotlieb (Ed.) *Social Networks and Social Support*. Beverly Hills: Sage, 1981.
3. Bennett, R. (Ed.). *Aging, isolation and resocialization*. Van Nostrand Reinhold Company, New York, New York, 1980.
4. Gordon, T. *Parent effectiveness training*. Wyden, New York, New York, 1970.
5. Harris, J. and Bodden, J. An activity group experience for disengaged elderly persons. *Journal of Gerontology*, 1978, *25*, 325-330.
6. Larson, R. Thirty years of research on the subjective well-being of older Americans. *Journal of Gerontology*, 1978, *33*, 109-125.
7. Lewis, M. and Butler, R. Life-review therapy: Putting memories to work in individual and group psychotherapy. *Geriatrics*, 1974, *29*, 199-205.
8. Lowenthal, M. and Boler, D. Voluntary vs. involuntary withdrawal. *Journal of Gerontology*, 1965, *20*, 363-371.
9. Lowenthal, M. and Havens, C. Interaction and adaptation: Intimacy as a critical variable. *American Sociological Review*, 1968, *33*, 20-31.
10. Mitchell, R. E. and Trickett, E. J. Task Force Report: Social networks as mediators of social support. *Community Mental Health Journal*, 1980, *16*, 27-44.
11. Mulligan, M. and Bennett, R. Assessment of mental health and social problems during multiple friendly visits: The development and evaluation of a friendly visitor program for

the isolated elderly. *International Journal of Aging and Human Development*, 1977, *8*, 43-65.

12. Peaco, D. Effectiveness of paraprofessional volunteers in friendly visting programs for the homebound elderly. Unpublished manuscript University of Missouri-St. Louis, 1980.

13. Pincus, A. Reminiscence in aging and its implications for social work practice. *Social Work*, 1970, *15*, 47-53.

14. Reinke, B., Holmes, D. and Denney, N. Influence on "friendly visitor" program on the cognitive functioning and morale of elderly persons. *American Journal of Community Psychology*, 1981, *9*, 491-504.

15. Rosen, C. and Rosen, S. Evaluating an intervention program for the elderly. *Community Mental Health Journal*, 1982, *18*, 21-23.

16. Weiner, M. The short-term effects of a resocialization program on the functioning of isolated, community-based geriatric patients, in *Aging, Isolation, and Resocialization*, R. Bennett (Ed.).

17. Wood, V., Wylie, M. and Sheafer, B. An analysis of a short self-report measure of life satisfaction: Correlation with rather judgments. *Journal of Gerontology*, 1966, *24*, 465-469.

Church-Based Programs
for Black Care-Givers
of Non-Institutionalized Elders

David Haber, PhD

ABSTRACT. Two hundred and eighty-two caregivers graduated from a 12-hour caregiving program conducted at eight church sites. The graduates reported more efficiency with performing caregiving activities but, in comparison to a control group, did not expand to new caregiving activities nor to linkages with formal service agencies. At the termination of the training program, mutual help groups were fostered at three church sites, and sustained to the present time—one year later. The mutual help groups have instituted senior watch programs, newsletters, fund-raisers, seminars, resource directories and health screenings. At one church site three neighboring churches cooperated on both the training program and the mutual help group.

INTRODUCTION

Caregiving for Non-Institutionalized Black Elders

As a population, Americans continue to grow older. The percentage of Americans over age 65 has tripled during this century, from 4% of the population at the turn of the century to 11% by 1980. The projection for the age segment 65 and over for the year 2020, when the baby boom cohort of 1950 becomes the gerontology boom cohort, is up to 20% of the population.

However, even more dramatic than the aging of Americans will be the "aging of the aged." For instance, while 1% of Americans today are age 85 and over, 4% will join the ranks of the very old by the

David Haber, Program Specialist, Institute of Gerontology, University of the District of Columbia, 1100 Harvard Street, N.W., Washington, D.C. 20009.

Funded by Administration on Aging's Model Projects and Demonstration Program, Award # 90AM0028/01.

year 2020 (Barrow & Smith, 1983). This growth is accompanied by a startling increase in vulnerability, including physical and mental frailty, as well as dependence on long-term care institutions, or family caregivers in the community. The option of long-term care institutions, however, is limited for black families. For example, while blacks constitute 11% of the national population, only 6% of all older persons residing in nursing homes are non-white (Soldo, 1977). The likely factors contributing to this inequity include institutional discrimination (Butler, 1975), shorter longevity (Jackson, 1980), and differences in the number of children who can share the caregiving burden (Soldo & DeVita, 1978). In this last regard, 35% of older, ever-married blacks had given birth to four or more children in 1970, compared to 27% of white older females.

Perhaps due to more reliance on family caregivers in the community, black elders have higher expectations toward family responsibility to older persons than do older whites (Seelbach & Sauer, 1977). It appears, however, that both expectations and actual responsibility for caring for the old are associated with low morale. Seelbach and Sauer (1977), for instance, report a correlation between expectation of filial responsibility and low morale, particularly among black families. Similarly, a five year longitudinal study by Robinson and Thurnher (1979) concludes that the actual responsibility of caring for older parents by their families is associated with low morale.

The Black Church as a Site for Program Intervention

During the 1970s there was a surge in religiosity that cut across all sectors of the American population, though the religiosity of black Americans continued to be stronger than it was for Americans in general (Gallup, 1977). Proportionately, more blacks were members of churches and attendance rates were higher.

Furthermore, census counts have underestimated the number of black church members. For instance, a higher percentage of black church members attend small, evangelical, storefront churches like the Spiritualist and Pentecostal churches, or Muslim sects, which typically go uncounted. Also, a number of blacks, particularly those in the Catholic denomination, go uncounted because of their existing membership in white churches.

Some social analysts suggest that racial discrimination is a distinguishing factor in the intensity of the religious behavior of black church members (Dancy, 1977). Blacks are under-represented in professional organizations, social clubs and other alternative sources of recognition and emotional satisfaction. Instead, the black church takes on many of the social functions that are performed by a variety of non-religious organizations in the white community.

Another reason that blacks turn to the church is the need for social services that are perceived to be unavailable through service agencies or philanthropic organizations. These organizations are frequently large, bureaucratic in structure, and located outside of the minority neighborhood. In contrast, the life space of the low-income minority family is rooted in the narrow locale of neighborhood, which typically includes the neighborhood church.

Historically, the black church plays an important role in strengthening the family and providing social services. Dancy, with a focus on the black elder, notes:

> A strong orientation toward religion and the black church is a cultural attribute which holds a great deal of importance in the lives of the black elderly.... The church is a channel through which a large segment of the black elderly can be reached.... When vital social services were not available to its parishioners, the black church provided the needed counsel, the services, the framework of meaning (1977).

An empirical study by Cantor and Mayer (1978) lends further support to the importance of the church for the older person:

> Religious institutions, according to the study data, play an important part in the lives of many inner city elderly, particularly black and Spanish respondents. It is not unexpected, therefore, that the third most frequently turned to source of assistance was religious leaders.

Another study by Cantor (1975) reports that attending church together is one of three activities that are most likely to engage older persons in socialization, including the older caregiver who needs respite from caring for a frail spouse. In fact, while organizational membership is very low for the inner city elderly, the highest proportion of membership by far (20%) is with elderly in a church or synagogue group (Cantor, 1978).

During the past half century, the social service orientation of the black church has grown stronger. Congregation members are less frequently oriented exclusively to other-worldly exhortation and emotional catharsis. Conversely, the Martin Luther King era produced increasing attention to social action and social justice. Since the early 1970s a growing number of black churches have begun to emphasize social service programs as part of their organizational mandate (Lincoln, 1974; Rathbone-McCuan & Hashimi, 1982).

Mutual Help Groups

The mutual help group idea began at least as far back as the mutual aid societies in the black churches in the 1700s. These societies were precursors to the modern version of a mutual help group. The first society was organized in 1787 in Philadelphia and was called the Free African Society. The purpose of this church-affiliated help group was to provide mutual assistance in times of sickness and other critical need. By the late 1800s there were nine mutual aid societies in Atlanta alone, and 6 were connected with churches (Frazier & Lincoln, 1974).

The modern prototype of a mutual help group is probably the Alcoholics Anonymous organization which began in the mid-1930s. This group, and the ones to follow, were created because of the lack of available professional or governmental assistance, and the inadequacy of existing informal help networks. In addition, the mutual help group is unique in its ability to create a personal, intimate, face-to-face atmosphere where persons of similar interest and experience can exchange ideas and coping techniques. Professional expertise, while it is obtained as needed, is secondary to the leadership of the lay membership.

It is now estimated that there are a half million mutual help groups in America, representing more than 15 million persons. The groups represent a tremendous array of interests, including nearly every disease category listed by the World Health Organization (Katz & Bender, 1976; Gartner & Riessman, 1977). Mutual help groups now provide more continuous care for chronic disease and disabilities than all the professional resources currently available in this country.

The application of mutual help groups to the needs of caregivers and noninstitutionalized elders has been noted by Haber (1983). In the specific area of caregiving for older adults, the number of mutual help groups has been growing rapidly. For instance, in the New Jersey Self-Help Sourcebook (1983) the following organizations have been listed: Caregivers for the Aging, Livingroom (Support for Relatives of the Elderly), Women with Aging Parents, Children of Aging Parents, Adult Children with Aging Parents, SHARE (Self-Help for Adults with Relatives who are Elderly, CAP (Caretakers of Aging Parents), etc.

Church-Based Programs: Training Program and Mutual Help Group

The 12-hour training program implemented by the Institute of Gerontology at the University of the District of Columbia is designed to introduce a variety of useful topics to church members who care for non-institutionalized elders. The training manual is adapted from the manual developed at the Institute of Gerontology at the University of Michigan-Wayne State University, entitled, *As Parents Grow Older: A Manual for Program Replication* (Silverman et al., 1981). The content of this manual has been restructured into seven topics, with each of the first six topics presented in one and a half hour classes, and the final topic in a three hour class. The seven topics are as follows:

1. Understanding the Psychological Aspects of Aging
2. Sensory Deprivation
3. Chronic Illnesses and Behavioral Changes with Age
4. Basic Nursing Care Skills for Care of the Patient at Home
5. Improving Communication
6. Living Arrangements and Shared Decision Making
7. Availability and Utilization of Community Resources

The idea of creating a mutual help group for caregivers is fostered throughout the 12-hour training program. Trainees are made aware of the tremendous flexibility of a mutual help group. For instance, existing church clubs can take on a new objective that includes a mutual help group for caregivers; or a new group can get started. Also, the functions of a mutual help group can be focused on one or more directions. For example, some groups emphasize meeting on an ongoing, regularly scheduled basis to share ideas, support and techniques of interest to elders in need and/or their caregivers. Some groups may implement a newsletter to provide useful information on caregiving or gerontological topics. Yet other groups may periodically invite outside experts to conduct seminars on topics of particular interest to church members. Finally, mutual help group members can be trained to use a comprehensive Resource Directory in order to make services and resources in the community available to all church members in need.

Whatever direction a mutual help group takes, its fundamental purpose is to continue the educational and resource-sharing goals of the training program, without dependency on professionals or funding agencies.

METHOD

Sample

Eight church sites from the District of Columbia were selected (with three neighboring churches participating at one church site) with three objectives guiding the selection process:

1. to represent the percentage of black churches within each of the major denominations in America,
2. to reflect as much diversity as the inner city of the District of Columbia will allow, in terms of income and educational level, size of congregation, percentage of membership who are elderly, and amount of church involvement with social services, and
3. to select churches with enthusiastic pastors and church leaders.

Thus, we selected three Baptist church sites, one African Methodist, one Methodist and one Episcopal site, plus two comparison sites which were Baptist. The comparison sites received the training program after the posttest interviews were completed.

Two hundred and eighty-two trainees graduated from the caregiving training programs, with 95 completing pretest and posttest interviews. Since the rapport with church members took precedence over the generalizability of the findings, we did not sample the 34% of the trainees who completed the interviews. Instead, we interviewed only those persons who volunteered to do the two interviews, and were willing to complete them at a selected church site during a designated interview period. Sixty-one respondents completed the training program prior to the posttest interview, with 25 (41%) participating in at least one mutual help group meeting. Thirty-four respondents attended the comparison churches, and completed the training program after the posttest interview. Of the 95 respondents, 99% were black and 87% female. The mean age was 56 years, with 50% retirees. Respondents were mostly lower income, very religious, and all could identify at least one person to whom they provided caregiving assistance. Any person who provided any type of self-defined caregiving assistance was eligible for the caregiving program.

Among the care recipients who received assistance from the caregiving respondents, 49 completed pretest and posttest interviews. The average age of the care recipients was 74 years, with a mean annual income of $5,000. Respondents were primarily black females with less than a high school education. The majority of the respondents were widowed, but only 14% lived alone. Care recipients were mainly retirees on social security. Half retired from service work, either maid or janitorial work, while 13% were retired professionals.

Administration of Instruments

The measurement instrument used for the interviews with caregivers was an amalgam of several existing instruments to assess caregiving behaviors and attitudes. One of these instruments, the OARS (Duke University, 1978), was the primary instrument administered to the care recipients as well.

The pretest interviews were conducted in March-April, 1982, and the posttest interviews in September-October, 1982. The original intent was to assess the impact of the 12-hour caregiving training program and the subsequent mutual help group meetings. However, organizational activities at the participating churches during the summer months of June, July and August were suspended until the Fall. Thus, on the average, the trainees who had joined mutual help groups were only able to attend two mutual help group meetings prior to the posttest interview.

Consequently, two separate sections for results will be reported: 1) the findings of the pretest and posttest interviews, which basically assess the impact of the training program, and 2) a documentation of the mutual help group activities after one year of existence.

Results of the Caregiving Training Program

Hypothesis One: Treatment caregivers will increase the quantity of caregiving activities in comparison to control caregivers.

The following caregiving activities were provided by at least one-third of the caregiving respondents: companionship (56%), transportation (49%), continual supervision or checking (47%), homemaker/household help (38%) and assistance with crime or safety precautions (34%). At the time of the posttest interview there was little change in the priority of caregiving activities noted above, nor were new caregiving activities undertaken. Among the 61 trainee-respondents there were only three reported instances of linkages with formal agency providers that were a result of information gained from the training program (see Table 1).

From a testimonial perspective, there were 88 separate comments on how the training program, the first few mutual help group meetings or the interview itself led to more efficient caregiving activity, or more effort at caregiving activity. However, there were no objective or quantitative measures to verify these testimonials.

Hypothesis Two: Treatment caregivers will have more positive attitudes toward caregiving in comparison to control caregivers.

The life satisfaction index, the caregiving satisfaction index, and the questionnaire items on intergenerational living, governmental versus family responsibility for the health needs of older persons, and attitudes toward placing an older relative in a nursing home were unchanged over time. This consistency over time was due to the unexpectedly positive attitudes reported during the pretest, with 85% of the caregivers reporting that their caregiving activities involved no sacrifice whatsoever, or a minor sacrifice.

Hypothesis Three: Treatment care recipients will improve physical/mental capacities and social resources in comparison to control care recipients.

The five rating scales of the OARS instrument: social resources, economic resources, mental health, physical health and activities of daily living, as well as the cumulative impairment score for all five scales, remained consistent over time for both treatment and control care recipients. Also, care recipients in general reported that they

Table 1.

Percentage of caregivers engaged in Specific Services

Type of Service		pretest	posttest	difference
homemaker	treatment	38	40	+2
	control	22	18	-2
employment	treatment	2	2	0
	control	1	2	+1
transportation	treatment	49	47	-2
	control	20	19	-1
home repairs	treatment	20	18	-2
	control	9	10	+1
social/recreational programs	treatment	18	16	-2
	control	7	4	-3
contact agencies	treatment	14	14	0
	control	6	7	+1
personal care	treatment	16	20	+4
	control	13	10	-3
nursing capacity	treatment	14	14	0
	control	14	9	-5
physical therapy/exercise	treatment	17	13	-4
	control	9	6	-3
counseling	treatment	17	17	0
	control	8	6	-2
financial/legal advice	treatment	26	26	0
	control	18	18	0
companionship	treatment	55	62	+6
	control	30	28	-2
crime or safety precautions	treatment	34	22	-12
	control	14	15	+1
reduced rates	treatment	17	17	0
	control	6	8	+2
meals at home/nutrition site	treatment	14	17	+3
	control	7	7	0
continual checking	treatment	47	46	-1
	control	25	23	-2
relocation	treatment	1	4	+3
	control	2	2	0
other	treatment	2	8	+6
	control	2	4	+2

received the same amount of caregiving assistance, and they received help from the same number of caregivers over time.

Results of the Mutual Help Groups

At the six treatment church sites, half were successful with sustaining a mutual help group over one year, with only occasional consultation from staff of the Institute of Gerontology at the University of the District of Columbia. Two of these churches had the highest socioeconomic status levels, and one church (actually the cluster of three churches that met at one church site) had the lowest socioeconomic status level. The following new caregiving activities were initiated by the three mutual help groups, with the cluster initiating the most activities:

1. A Senior Watch program to make sure that homes are not lost through unpaid taxes, utilities, etc.
2. Newsletters related to gerontological or caregiving activities.
3. Lectures on wills and pre-paid funeral arrangements, with efforts to make sure that all church members are prepared for the event of death.
4. Fund-raisers to support church projects, i.e., the mutual help group newsletters, a ramp for seniors and the handicapped, etc.
5. Lectures on issues of concern, such as housing for seniors, transportation, community services and resources, etc.
6. A resource directory for all church members, with designated members who coordinate its use, and update it.
7. Health screenings organized at the church sites.

Discussion and Conclusions

In general, persons who completed the training program did not increase the scope of their caregiving activities, nor improve their attitudes over time. This result was not surprising given the sample of respondents who were not burdened by their caregiving role at the time of the pretests. Furthermore, the inability to establish the mutual help groups prior to the posttest interviews eliminated from analysis a potentially powerful influence on caregiving behaviors and attitudes.

The consistency of physical and mental capacities and social resources of the care recipients were also affected by the same factors. There did not seem to be a substantial amount of stress in the caregiver-care receiving relationship at the time of the pretest interview, and a brief, 12-hour training program is not a particularly powerful vehicle for changing years of established behaviors and attitudes.

The most successful part of the project appeared to be the mutual help groups, and yet only half the groups were able to sustain regularly scheduled activities for more than a year after the professional leadership had left the church site. The most important factor for implementing and sustaining a mutual help group was the enthusiasm, commitment and ability of the pastor and/or church leaders to organize and motivate church members. At the three church sites where mutual help groups were not initiated or sustained, the initial enthusiasm of the church pastor or deaconesses quickly waned.

In terms of predicting the success of the mutual help groups, no factor other than leadership appeared to be relevant. The three successful church sites were not homogeneous in terms of denomination, size of church membership, history of social service activity, percentage of membership that is elderly, and socioeconomic status. Conversely, at all three church sites that were successful at implementing mutual help groups, the church pastors remained involved with the caregiving activities, the deaconesses continued their enthusiastic support, and at least one church member kept in contact with a staff member at the Institute of Gerontology to discuss concerns and recent accomplishments.

In brief, the project findings stimulated several conclusions with implications for program administrators and policy-makers:

1. The mutual help groups were successful with initiating multiple projects, involving hundreds of church members. Future research efforts should focus on this aspect of intervention, with less attention to the impact of a short-term training program, except as it relates to fostering the emergence of a mutual help group.

2. The investigation of mutual help groups will be difficult, given the overreliance on testimonials in the past, and the scarcity of objective and quantifiable efforts. Future studies should consider why caregivers do, or do not, join a mutual help group; the type of community site which fosters the emergence of a group; short-term and long-term assessments; control groups; triangulated assessment techniques like obser-

vation, interview, questionnaire and/or informants; and the impact of the mutual help group on the care recipients as well as the caregiving participants.

3. The most successful mutual help group in terms of the number of projects it initiated, involved the cluster of three churches operating at a single community site. This type of cooperation, or friendly competition, among churches may spur greater accomplishments than would occur with one church at its own site. Further exploration is needed on caregiving programs that are based on organizational frameworks that are ecumenical, interfaith, or a cluster of churches within a single denomination.

4. This project was one of the few studies of caregiving to focus on a non-service-agency-utilizing population (Horowitz & Dobrof, 1982). While it is important for some studies to examine caregiving families before they reach a service agency, it might be more productive to target families that are experiencing a sense of caregiving burden or sacrifice, in contrast to this study's sample population.

5. The training program was not successful with fostering new caregiving activities, nor linkages with formal service providers, except on a very limited basis. As the "aging of the aged" continues, more alternatives need to be explored for linking informal caregivers who are not willing to join a mutual help group to formal service providers.

REFERENCES

Barrow, G., and P. Smith, *Aging, Ageism and Society*, end. ed., West Publishing Company, N.Y: 1983.

Butler, R., *Why Survive? Being Old in America*, Harper & Row Publishers, Inc., N.Y: 1975.

Cantor, M., "Life Space and the Social Support System of the Inner City Elderly of New York City," *The Gerontologist*, 1975, 15, 23-27.

Cantor, M., "The Informal Support System of the "Family Less" Elderly—Who Takes Over?" presented at 31st Annual Scientific Meeting of the Gerontological Society of America, Dallas, Texas, November 18, 1978.

Cantor, M., and M. Mayer, "Factors in Differential Utilization of Services by Urban Elderly," *Journal of Gerontological Social Work*, 1978, 1, 1, 47-62.

Dancy, J. Jr., *The Black Elderly*. Institute of Gerontology, University of Michigan-Wayne State University, Michigan: 1977.

Duke University, *The OARS Methodology: Multidimensional Functional Assessment*, 2nd. ed., Center for the Study of Aging and Human Development, Durham, North Carolina: 1978.

Frazier, E., and C. Lincoln, *The Negro Church in America/The Black Church Since Frazier*, Schocken Books, Inc., N.Y: 1974.

Gartner, A., and F. Riessman, *Self-Help in the Human Services*, Jossey-Bass Publishers, San Francisco: 1977.

Haber, D., "Mutual Help Groups Among Older Persons," *The Gerontologist*, 1983, 23, 3, 251-253.

Horowitz, A., and R. Dobrof, "The Role of Families in Providing Long-Term Care to the Frail and Chronically Ill Elderly Living in the Community," Final Report submitted to the Health Care Financing Administration, DHHS, May, 1982.

Jackson, J., *Minorities and Aging*, Wadsworth Publishing Co., California: 1980.

Katz, A., and E. Bender, *The Strength in Us*, New Viewpoints, New York: 1976.

Lincoln, C., *The Black Church Since Frazier*, Schocken Books, N.Y.: 1974.

New Jersey Self-Help Sourcebook, Self-Help Clearinghouse, St. Clare's Community Mental Health Center, Denville, New Jersey: 1983.

Silverman, A. et al., *As Parents Grow Older: A Manual for Program Replication*, Institute of Gerontology, University of Michigan, Ann Arbor: 1981.

Soldo, B., "Accounting for Racial Differences in Institutional Placements," paper presentation at the Gerontological Society of American Meeting, November, 1977.

Soldo, B., and C. DeVita, "Profiles of Black Aged," Workshop paper, Conference on Blacks and Retirement, Washington, D.C., February 2-5, 1978.

Agency-Family Partnerships: Case Management of Services for the Elderly

Marsha Mailick Seltzer, PhD
Kathryn Simmons, MSW
Joann Ivry, MSW
Leon Litchfield, MSW

ABSTRACT. This paper describes a research and demonstration project in which partnerships are formed between agency social workers and family members of elderly clients. While the social worker retains responsibility for counseling and provision of support to the elderly client, the family member is taught by the social worker to assume responsibility for the case management of services provided to his/her elderly relative.

Practice issues which have emerged during the first year of this three-year project include: the generalizability of findings in light of the special characteristics of agency clients, the definition of the agency-family partnership, confidentiality in the context of this partnership, exceptions to family involvement, clients without families, and our experiences with research-practice collaboration. Each of these issues is discussed in this paper.

Currently, social agencies which serve the elderly are faced with the prospect of substantially increased client needs, as the number and proportion of elderly persons in our population rises. As people live longer, their need for basic support—economic, emotional,

Marsha Mailick Seltzer and Leon Litchfield are affiliated with Boston University School of Social Work, 264 Bay State Road, Boston, MA 02215. Kathryn Simmons and Joann Ivry are affiliated with Jewish Family and Children's Services, Boston, Massachusetts.

The project described in this paper received support from the Permanent Charities Fund of Boston, the Blanchard Foundation (managed by the Boston Safe Deposit and Trust Company), the Ratchesky Foundation, and the Fox Memorial Fund. We are grateful to Rose Ann Ariel, Renee Hecht, and Elaine Mittell for their invaluable data collection efforts and to Joseph Bronstein, Simon Krakow, Richard Levin, Louis Lowy, and Mildred Mailick for their critique of an earlier version of this manuscript.

and functional—increases. At the same time, social service agencies must cope with constant or shrinking resources. This paper presents one strategy for improving social services for elderly clients, namely the involvement of family members of elderly clients of a social services agency as partners with the social worker in the case management of services to the elderly individual. The purpose of this paper is to report on a number of social work practice issues that have emerged in the course of our experiences with family involvement.

LITERATURE REVIEW

There is increasing concensus in the gerontological and social work literatures that it is desirable to support and involve the family of elderly clients. Hartman (1981) recently proposed that the family should be recognized as the primary social service institution, and Silverman and Brahce (1979) asserted that "the family is now considered to be the most important agency supporting the elderly" (p. 79). Monk (1981) went even further by stating that: "it is the function of social workers to...mobilize kin networks so that they take responsibility for those in the family" (p. 63).

There is widespread agreement among gerontologists that the family is often the basis of security for adults in later life (e.g., Lowy, 1977; Shanas, 1961; Callahan, Diamond, Giele & Morris, Note 1). As pointed out by Collins and Pancoast (1976), "were it not for the informal services of helping networks, social agencies...would be swamped. Besides carrying the bulk of the service load in many sectors...helping networks also carry out a widespread preventive program. They offer accessible, individualized services formal agencies could never match" (p. 25). Despite the decline of the three generational family in the U.S., meaningful family linkages can and do occur extensively. The family serves as a voluntary yet primary deliverer of material and affective support to the elderly (Sussman, 1965, 1976). As well, a number of studies have found a similar involvement of family with the disabled and/or chronically ill elderly, a particularly difficult segment of the elderly population (Brody, Poulschock, & Masciocchi, 1978; Shanas, Townsend, Wedderburn, Friis, Milhoj, & Stehouwer, 1968; Shanas & Maddox, 1976).

Less has been written about the role of friends and neighbors as sources of informal support. The limited data that are available suggest that the involvement of non-relatives in the informal support system is considerable, and that this often is a reciprocal arrangement (Atchley, 1980; Cantor, 1979; Lopata, 1975; Lowenthal & Robinson, 1976; Rosow, 1967; Sherman, 1975, Gore, Note 2; Morris, Sherwood, Kasten, & Miranda, Note 3).

When elderly persons need agency-based services, the role of the family in providing support to the elderly relative is not clear. As Shanas and Sussman (1977) have noted, there are no precise guidelines regarding who is in charge of coordinating the case of an elderly client—the elderly person him or herself, the family, or the formal service worker. Smyer (1980) noted "...there are certain functions which families perform better and certain tasks which are more appropriately the responsibility of society. At the current time, however, there is little information about the best collaboration between these two" (p. 254). The purpose of the research and demonstration project described in this paper is to determine whether family members (or non-family helpers) can be involved as partners with the social service agency, and if so, whether this involvement has a favorable effect on the elderly client and on the family. Specifically, the project entails training family members to function as case managers for their elderly relatives.

Case management has emerged in recent years as an attractive concept with which to respond to a fragmented and complicated service delivery system (Austin, 1983; Brody, 1979; Intagliata, 1982; Monk, 1981; Wylie & Austin, 1978, Beatrice, Note 4). Case management is a service coordination mechanism designed to provide multiple services to clients with complex needs. Among the activities included in the case management function are: screening, assessment, case planning, service arrangement, service provision, service monitoring, linkage, and reassessment. The essence of the case management approach is to establish responsibility for services within a single locus of control. Service control is retained by the case manager who acts as consultant and facilitator, integrates and individualizes services, and establishes a personal relationship with the client.

While case management is a legitimate professional social work function, it is also performed by para-professionals and, as Sussman (1977) has written, by family members as well. Additionally, as

Monk (1981) noted, given the dramatic increase in life expectancy, it is unrealistic to expect that there will be enough social workers available to coordinate services for an expanded aged population. Furthermore, and perhaps most important, it is debatable whether the professionalization of services such as case management is necessary or even advisable. Cantor, Rehr, and Trotz (1981) argue that "there is no question...that case management is and should continue to be a basic responsibility of the informal support system—a family member in particular" (p. 568).

In the design of agency and family roles in the delivery of services to the elderly, it may be most appropriate for social workers to channel some of their expertise into strengthening the family's helping and case management capacities and serving as a trainer and consultant to the family. The project that is described in the discussion which follows is an attempt to operationalize Cantor et al's (1981) above argument along these lines.

FAMILY-CENTERED COMMUNITY CARE FOR THE ELDERLY

The Jewish Family and Children's Services (JFCS) of Boston and the Boston University School of Social Work have collaborated on the development and implementation of the Family-Centered Community Care for the Elderly Project. The goal of this intervention is to utilize, strengthen, and enhance family capacities so that ultimately the agency's role in case management can be reduced. Specifically, since January 1, 1982, new elderly clients of JFCS have been randomly assigned to two groups: innovative family involvement (the experimental group) and traditional family involvement (the control group). When an elderly client is assigned to the experimental group, an attempt is made to involve the client's family (or a non-family helper) as a partner with the social worker, specifically in the role of case manager. In the control group, no such special effort is made to involve the family in the process of planning and monitoring the services provided by the social worker. Instead, the traditional approach to service delivery is employed. As part of the traditional approach, the family may or may not be involved, depending upon the interest and judgment of the social worker, the client, and the family member.

It should be noted that the partnership that is proposed here is distinct from traditional forms of family involvement. Casework with elderly clients and families has always aimed to involve families. Partnership, however, involves the integration of the formal and informal support systems in sharing *responsibility* for the coordination of services to the elderly person. While the professional literature is full of exhortation to professionals and agencies to foster strong links with families and to strengthen the interface of the formal and informal support networks, very few articles present concrete practice guidelines for developing partnerships in which responsibility is shared between agency personnel and family members.

Family-Centered Community Care for the Elderly defines partnership as the mutual sharing of responsibility between the agency and the family in planning for the case management of services to the elderly. Many family members in fact are already providing case management services for their relatives and many more could be assisted to do so. In this demonstration project, social workers in the experimental group introduce a series of interventions designed to maximize the family's ability to assume responsibility for formal service planning and monitoring. Such interventions are not used with the control group. This experimental intervention includes four components:

1. the *expectation* that the family will assume some case management responsibility.
2. *collaboration* between the family member and the social worker as true partners on the development of the client's service plan.
3. the provision to the family of *informational manuals* which include information about entitlements, strategies for locating and utilizing resources, and descriptions of federal, state and private programs for the elderly. Five informational manuals have been developed for this project on the following topics:
   —In-Home Services and Nutrition
   —Housing, Day Care Centers, Respite Care, and Nursing Homes
   —Transportation and Social Opportunities
   —Financial Entitlement and Legal Protective Services
   —Advocacy
4. *regular meetings* and/or telephone contacts between the family member and the social worker to discuss the case manage-

ment needs of the elderly person, to assign tasks, to monitor the completion of case management tasks, to monitor the provision of services, and to identify additional problems that warrant attention. These contacts occur at least bi-weekly.

Both experimental and control group clients and their families are systematically assessed periodically during the course of service. Specifically, the elderly clients are assessed at intake with respect to their background characteristics, health status, functional abilities, cognitive and emotional status, formal services received, and extent of informal support. In addition, interviews are conducted with family members.[1] Following the completion of service, both experimental and control group clients are re-assessed in order to determine the extent to which they have changed in functioning and in status since the intake assessment. In addition, an assessment is conducted of the extent of family involvement in providing support to the elderly client and in assuming case management responsibilities.

The purpose of the control group in this study is to provide an indication of how the members of the experimental group (and their families) would have functioned had they not received the intervention. Simply observing change over time in experimental group clients and their families is not a sufficiently rigorous research design for our purposes. One reason that a control group is necessary in gerontological research is that there are times when deterioration is observed in an elderly person's functioning as part of the natural course of events. Without a control group with which to compare the experimental group, any deterioration in the experimental group could be mistakenly interpreted to indicate negative effects of the intervention.

The control group is also important when examining the effect of the intervention on the families. Most families perform some case management task for their elderly relatives, without the benefit of any special agency involvement. The question examined in this demonstration effort is whether the experimental intervention can

---

[1] Whereas all experimental group family members are interviewed at intake, only half of the control group family members are interviewed at that point in service. We have some concern that the interview itself may have the effect of increasing family involvement, and therefore we plan to conduct a comparison between control group cases whose family members are interviewed and those whose family members are not interviewed.

raise the level of family involvement beyond where it would have been in the absence of this intervention. The control group provides the estimate of the extent to which experimental families would have performed case management responsibilities had they not been trained. Thus, the impact of the Family-Centered Community Care for the Elderly project will be observable in the difference between experimental and control group clients in their level of functioning at case closing and in the extent and type of involvement on the part of their family members throughout the intervention. Specifically, by comparing the experimental with the control groups, it will be possible to determine whether the innovative family involvement makes a difference with respect to the following eight outcomes:

1. the extent to which the families of elderly clients actually are involved in the planning and monitoring of services delivered to their elderly relatives (i.e., the extent to which they assume case management functions);
2. the strength of the informal support network of the elderly clients;
3. the number and types of services planned for and delivered to the clients;
4. the rate of institutionalization and other measures of residential stability (e.g., number of moves)
5. the functional abilities of the elderly clients;
6. the extent to which elderly clients feel that they can rely on their relatives for support;
7. the level of satisfaction of the relative with agency services; and
8. the amount of time agency social workers spend on each case.

During the first year of this two-year research and demonstration project, 47 clients and their families have participated in the experimental group and 50 in the control group. An additional 100 cases are anticipated during the second year of the project. Analysis of the effects of this intervention will be conducted following the completion of the second year. To date, data analysis has focused on the descriptive characteristics of the clients and their families at intake and their residential status at case closing.

In the design and implementation of this project and in the preliminary analysis of data, a number of issues have emerged which have provoked considerable thought and discussion among project personnel. These are discussed below.

CHARACTERISTICS OF AGENCY CLIENTS

One issue that warrants examination pertains to the extent to which those elderly persons who use the Jewish Family and Children's Service are representative of the general population of older adults. This issue has implications for the generalizability of our findings. Several differences are apparent between JFCS clients and the general population of elderly persons. For one, nearly all project clients are Jewish. Another difference is in the extent of involvement of the informal support system. To date, only 5% of those families in the experimental group who have been approached to become partners with agency workers were unwilling to collaborate with the social worker in the assessment, planning and monitoring of the older client's case management needs. We expected that the need for agency involvement would be highest when family involvement was at a minimum. We were thus surprised to find that the elderly clients who utilize this agency are those who have an active, informal support system. Replication of this project with other samples—particularly with other ethnic groups—is therefore a priority for future research.

Another area of difference is in the age of the clients. Nationally, the mean age of the elderly (those aged 65+) is estimated to be about 75.[2] During the first year of our project, clients averaged 80 years of age (range = 59 to 93). Fully 26% were over age 85.

Several other characteristics of this group of clients were found to be consistent with their advanced age. For example, although nationally, only 5% of the nation's elderly live in nursing homes, at case closing, 32% of the sample had moved from the community to nursing homes. In addition, project clients tend to be quite impaired in their functional, emotional and cognitive status. Whereas assessments of the general elderly population suggest that approximately 80% of the elderly are self-sufficient in their performance of activities of daily living (Branch & Jette, 1983; Tolliver, 1983), only 50% of project clients were found to be independent in this domain.

---

[2]This estimate was provided by the U.S. Census Bureau on the basis of preliminary analysis of 1980 census data.

Similarly, whereas 15% of the elderly are estimated to suffer from depression (Tolliver, 1983), fully 37% of project clients were judged by their social workers to be depressed. The project clients were also more impaired cognitively. Nationally, less than 10% of the elderly are disoriented or demented (Wershow, 1981), whereas 35% of project cases have some memory loss, and another 5% have severe memory loss.

In sum, our sample appears to be distinct from the cross-section of the elderly population in a number of respects. They are older, more frail, and more impaired than is typical of elderly persons, yet their families remain involved. These characteristics pose both unusual challenges and opportunities in our attempt to involve families as partners with the agency.

DEFINITION OF PARTNERSHIP

The involvement of family members as partners has required that we carefully conceptualize the meaning of partnership and operationalize it with respect to project procedures. One study that was helpful in clarifying the meaning of partnership more fully (Froland, Pancoast, Chapman, & Kimboko, 1981), presented the findings of a survey of the efforts of 30 agencies to form linkages with the informal support system. The authors described the difficulties inherent in such partnerships, as follows:

> An attempt to link formal and informal modes of support is likely to result in a clashing of two different cultures: one seeking the reliability of formal rules and routine procedures, the other emphasizing the privacy of unspoken rules and spontaneous activity. Norms of exchange, conceptions of problems and solutions, and beliefs about authority and responsibility are considerably different and potentially at odds (p. 24).

Froland and his colleagues identified three types of partnerships that have been developed by agencies in their work with family members: coordinative, collegial and directive. A coordinative relationship is characterized by "a relatively high degree of independent action in which helpers decide what they will work on, take more responsibility for tasks and activities and receive little or no supervision from agency staff" (p. 62). In a collegial relationship, "staff and helpers share the responsibility of deciding what is to be done (but) staff do not supervise or monitor helpers" (pp. 62-63). In a directive relationship, "staff systematically recruit helpers, often requiring a formal commitment from those selected. The helpers' activities are supervised and monitored" (p. 64).

In Family-Centered Community Care for the Elderly, the partnership that is formed between the social worker and the family member most closely parallels the directive relationship conceptualized by Froland et al. (1981) but also contains elements of their collegial-type relationship. The partnership is first formed when the social worker approaches the family member and obtains his/her agreement to participate. The social worker defines the focus and parameters of the partnership—case management activities—and the social worker trains the family member in selected case management tasks. The family member collaborates with the social worker in setting the case management agenda and, following training, he/she assume responsibility for the performance of at least one case management task. The social worker monitors the family member's work through bi-weekly contacts, either by telephone or in person, and provides support and continued training to the family as the need arises.

In sum, although the agency-family partnership in Family-Centered Community Care for the Elderly is not fully collegial, it is a true partnership nonetheless. While the social worker is directive, the partners work together in activities that have been identified as falling within the defined area of case management. Training is intended to empower the family member and to reduce his/her (and the elderly client's) dependency on the agency when needs arise in the future.

CONFIDENTIALITY

Training family members in the development of case management skills promotes a number of changes in the family-agency relationship. In traditional social work practice and in the control group, the family is seen as an extension of the client. In the experimental group, the elderly person is the client and the family is seen as a distinct resource. However, the partnership that emerges poses challenges for the maintenance of client/worker confidentiality in relation to family members.

The National Association of Social Workers Code of Ethics states: "The social worker should respect the privacy of clients and hold in confidence all information obtained in the course of professional service" (NASW, 1980). When a client agrees to have a family member assume a partnership role with the agency, is the need for maintaining the boundaries of confidentiality eliminated? Is the effectiveness of a partnership diffused if information is withheld from a partner? What answers should be given in response to clients' questions related to the content of conversations about them? What about family members' rights to information? For example, how does one respond to the brother asking "What did my mother say about our arguments?"

It is essential that a clear definition of the extent and the limits of the agency/family partnership be outlined at the beginning of the partnership. The contract that is made with the family at the outset is that the agency and family member join together for the purpose of developing and implementing a case management service plan. It is made clear that family access to the records is not a component of partnership and furthermore that the social worker alone provides the clinical counseling services, as needed, to the elderly client. It is the social worker's responsibility to carefully maintain the boundaries of confidentiality for both the family member and for the client. When questions arise which jeopardize this boundary, family members and elderly clients need to be redirected to one another, using the social worker as a liaison if needed.

EXCEPTIONS TO FAMILY INVOLVEMENT

Are there any instances in which encouraging the family to assume case management responsibilities for an elderly relative would have negative repercussions for the elderly person and/or for the family member? The literature suggests that middle-age adults often experience a "role-strain" (Miller, 1981; Monk, 1979; Zarit, 1980; Lowy, Note 5). When one is confronted with one's own aging and the competing demands of teenage children, career involvement, and aging parents, there is a struggle to balance these demands. The following case study illustrates this issue.

Mrs. W. was referred to JFCS by the home care agency supplying her homemaker. She was experiencing a reactive depression to her husband's recent death. For the last ten years, Mrs. W. had numerous medical problems and her husband assumed all responsibility for running the household. Mrs. W. now had these responsibilities thrust back on her and was trying to re-establish herself as an independent woman. Because of her numerous physical limitations, this was quite difficult. Mrs. W. designated her daughter, Barbara, as the family member to whom she felt closest. However, Barbara was also having problems.

One month prior to her father's death, Barbara's son had been killed in a freak accident. Barbara was dealing with her son's death as well as her father's. In addition, she had to be responsive to the reactions of her husband, daughter and mother to these losses, and her mother's increased dependency needs.

Was this a case in which it was appropriate to minimize the assumption of additional responsibility by the family member? While involving Barbara in the development and coordination of Mrs. W.'s service plan and supplying Barbara with the project training materials, the agency social worker supported her needs by temporarily assuming the case management tasks until she was better able to handle this responsibility. Also, her mother was well able to assume the case management of some of her own services. She gained a sense of mastery as she developed a new feeling of independence. Barbara limited her case management activity to weekly monitoring of the services provided and worked with her mother on the resolution of problems with services whenever that became necessary. The social worker worked with Mrs. W. on those unresolved grief issues related to her husband's death as well as to the loss of her grandson which had been immobilizing her. She also helped Mrs. W. to develop the necessary skills for case management. Both mother and daughter were pleased with the delineation of roles.

Another reason to minimize involvement is related to unique family dynamics, as is illustrated by the F. family.

Bernard had a very hostile-dependent relationship with his parents, who were the agency clients, and he had maintained some distance from them for the past five years. He felt that this break was necessary for his own emotional well-being. His father was not hospitalized and was being cared for in a nursing home. His mother, who remained in the community, had a long history of psychiatric problems and was now demanding more of Bernard's attention. Should the agency encourage the son's involvement with his mother? Should he be trained in case management skills?

The setting of clear limits was one of the keys in assisting Bernard and his mother, Mrs. F. Bernard agreed to help his mother to make a Medicaid application for his father, but he felt unable to take responsibility for the supervision of the services his mother received. The social worker therefore assumed these roles.

What is the minimum amount of case management responsibility that can be assumed by the family in order to qualify as a partner? In our project, the assumption of one new case management task is the minimum definition of partnership. The extent of the social worker's responsibility can thus range from nearly all of the case management required in a case to none at all if the family member assumes this role fully.

In sum, there are cases in which full partnership may not be advisable. Examples include instances when the family member is undergoing an acutely stressful period or has overwhelming ongoing responsibilities, when the family member is emotionally or cognitively unable to serve as a partner, when the elderly person and the family member are estranged from one another, and when the elderly person is unwilling to allow the family member to assume the role of partner. It is often the case that another family member can be identified who can more appropriately serve as the social worker's partner. However, keeping family involvement to a minimum might be necessary in selected cases. It is important to note that in the vast majority of cases, family involvement is not only possible but also desirable. As we indicated earlier, families have refused to join as partners with the agency in only 5% of the cases in which they are asked. Thus, lack of family involvement is the exception not the rule.

CLIENTS WITHOUT FAMILIES

As noted earlier in this paper, the literature suggests that when an elderly person does not have or is not in contact with primary family members, or when the family members live some distance from their elderly relative, friends make up the core of the older person's informal support system. In the absence of family, two questions arise: 1) are clients willing to ask friends to assume a partnership role with the agency, and 2) are friends willing to take on the responsibility of this role? Our experience during the first year of the project has been that there are very few instances (4 cases out of 97) in which friends are identified as primary sources of support. In no instance in which the elderly person had a relative was a friend identified instead. Thus, although the literature suggests that friends provide support to older adults—particularly in the area of instrumental activities of daily living—the elderly client appears not to expect friends to assume the more demanding responsibility of case management. It is possible that older adults are more comfortable receiving instrumental help from their friends, but are reluctant to become dependent upon them by allowing them to plan and monitor services on their behalf.

If friends are not a resource for case management responsibility, what are the alternatives? Our experience is that the social service agency assumes the function of case manager when family members are not available. Fully 75% of the case management needs of clients who had no identifiable family member were met by the agency social worker. Future investigations should examine whether it is desirable and feasible to involve other non-professionals and/or para-professionals (e.g., volunteers, case aides) as case managers when family are unavailable.

RESEARCH-PRACTICE COLLABORATION

In the Family-Centered Community Care for the Elderly project, social research and social work practice are integrated for the purpose of designing and evaluating the new service model of family-agency partnership in case management. The research component, which requires a substantial amount of data collection from the social workers, has been successfully integrated into the agency's day-to-day operation because the project has received clear support from the agency's administration and because the social work staff have been involved since the beginning of the project in the development of the research procedures.

Covey (1982) discussed a number of problems that may emerge when experiments are conducted about social programs. Among these are, problems with program goals and measurement, and the challenge of constructing an adequate control group. When planning the Family-Centered Community Care for the Elderly project, these and other issues were considered. The strategies that we developed for this project have to a large extent minimized such problems. For example, regarding the identification of goals, the top administration of the agency was instrumental in articulating the goals of the project, and regarding measurement, the project's social work staff was involved in the development and refinement of data collection instruments for use in measuring progress toward these goals.

Second, we have attempted to handle the problem of the construction of adequate control groups by randomly assigning elderly clients to either the experimental or the control group. Randomization is often resisted in social work agencies, either on ethical or practical grounds. In Family-Centered Community Care for the Elderly, the control group receives the same services they would have been given had the project not existed. Since services are not withheld, few questions have been articulated by the workers, the clients, or their families about the ethics of the control group. Also, we have minimized some of the practical problems associated with construction of an equivalent control group by randomly assigning cases to project workers after the intake process has been completed. Although initially we had some concern that there would be difficulty in having one worker take the initial call and another provide continuing service to a case, no problems with this procedure have emerged to date. Covey (1982) also discusses the problem of "contamination" of the control group by the experimental group. We have attempted to minimize this problem by holding separate staff and supervision meetings for experimental and control workers. However, contamination remains a possibility.

CONCLUSIONS

The project has attempted to design and formalize a role for family members of elderly clients which is complementary to the role of the social worker. The purpose of the intervention is to train family members in case management so that when new problems emerge in the lives of their elderly relatives, the family can respond more autonomously, thus minimizing their dependency on the agency. Although lessening some of the case management burden for social workers was not a primary objective of the intervention, it is the case that as family members assume some of these tasks, social workers can focus their efforts on activities which families cannot be expected to perform, such as counseling, handling more complex case management problems, and advocacy.

The process of engaging families, training them, and supporting them in the performance of case management responsibilities has been surprisingly smooth. As we noted, nearly all family members who have been approached have agreed to participate. Therefore, the first stage of the project—engaging the family—appears thus far to have been successful. Whether there will be a favorable impact on the elderly person or on the family has yet to be determined. These data will be analyzed shortly. Future research will examine the effectiveness of the family-centered intervention with other populations and will explore additional strategies for providing support to family members and engaging them as partners with social service agencies.

REFERENCE NOTES

1. Callahan, J. J., Diamond, L.D., Giele, J.Z., & Morris, R. *Responsibility of families for their severely disabled elders.* Waltham, Massachusetts: Brandeis University, 1979, mimeo.

2. Gore, S. *Influence of social support and related variables in ameliorating the consequences of job loss.* Unpublished dissertation, University of Pennsylvania, 1973.

3. Morris, J., Sherwood, S., Kasten, S., & Miranda, G. *The Parkview Towers' resident typology.* Boston: Hebrew Rehabilitation Center for Aged, 1979, mimeo.

4. Beatrice, D.F. *Case management: A policy option for long-term care.* University Health Policy Consortium, unpublished manuscript, Brandeis University, 1979.

5. Lowy, L. *The older generation: what is due, what is owed.* Paper presented at the SPSSI Symposium, APA Conference on the Prevention of Intergenerational Conflict in the Family, August 28, 1981.

REFERENCES

Atchley, R.C. *The social forces in later life.* Belmont, California: Wadsworth Publishing Company, 1980.

Austin, C.D. Case management in long-term care: Options and Opportunities. *Health and Social Work,* 1983, *8,* 16-30.

Branch, L.G., & Jette, A.M. Elders' use of informal long-term care assistance. *The Gerontologist,* 1983, *23,* 51-56.

Brody, E. Message from the president. *The Gerontologist,* 1979, *19,* 516.

Brody, S., Poulschock, S., & Masciocchi, C. The family caring unit: a major consideration in the long term support system. *The Gerontologist,* 1978, *18,* 6, 556-561.

Cantor, M. Neighbors and friends: An overlooked resource in the informal support system. *Research on Aging,* 1979, 1, 434-463.

Cantor, M., Rehr, H., & Trotz, V. Workshop II: Case management and family involvement. *The Mount Sinai Journal of Medicine*, 1981. *48*, 566-568.

Collins, A.H., & Pancoast, D.L. *Natural helping networks*. Washington, DC: NASW, 1976.

Covey, H.C. Basic problems of applying experiments to social programs. *Social Service Review*, 1982, *56*, 424-437.

Froland, C., Pancoast, D.L., Chapman, N.J., & Kimboko, P.J. *Helping networks and human services*. Beverly Hills: Sage Publications, 1981.

Hartman, A. The family: A central focus for practice. *Social Work*, 1981, *26*, 1, 7-13.

Intagliata, J. Improving the quality of community care for the chronically mentally disabled: The role of case management. *Schizophrenia Bulletin*, 1982, *8*, 655-674.

Lopata, H.Z. Support system of elderly urbanites: Chicago of the 1970's. *The Gerontologist*, 1975, *15*, 35-41.

Lowenthal, M.E., & Robinson, B. Social networks and isolation. In R.H. Binstock and E. Shanas (Eds.), *Handbook of aging and the social sciences*. New York: Van Nostrand Reinhold, 1976.

Lowy, L. Adult children and their parents: Dependency or dependability? *Long-term care and health services administration quarterly*, 1977, *1*, 243-248.

Miller, D.A. The sandwich generation: Adult children of the aging. *Social Work*, 1981, 419-423.

Monk, A. Family support in old age. *Social Work*, November 1979, *24*, 6, 533-38.

Monk, A. Social work with the aged: Principles of practice. *Social Work*, 1981, *26*, 1, 61-68.

National Association of Social Workers. *Code of Ethics*. Washington, DC: NASW, 1980.

Rosow, I. *Social integration of the aged*. New York: The Free Press, 1967.

Shanas, E. *Family relationships of older people*. Chicago: Health Information Foundations, 1961.

Shanas, E., & Maddox, G.L. Aging, health and the organization of health resources. In R.H. Binstock, & E. Shanas (Eds.), *Handbook of aging and the social sciences*. New York: Van Nostrand Reinhold Co., 1976.

Shanas, E., & Sussman, M.D. (Eds.). *Family, bureaucracy and the elderly*. Durham, N.C.: Duke University Press, 1977.

Shanas, E., Townsend, P., Wedderburn, D., Friis, H., Milhoj, P., & Stehouwer, J. *Old people in three industrial societies*. New York: Atherton Press, 1968.

Sherman, S.R. Mutual assistance and support in retirement housing. *Journal of Gerontology*, 1975, *30*, 479-83.

Silverman, A.G., & Brahce, C.I. As parents grow older: an intervention model. *Journal of Gerontological Social Work*, 1979, *2*, 1, 77-85.

Smyer, M.A. The differential usage of services by impaired elderly. *Journal of Gerontology*, 1980, *35*, 249-55.

Sussman, M.B. Relationships of adult children with their parents in the United States. In E. Shanas and G. Streib (Eds.), *Social structure and the family: Generational relations*. Englewood Cliffs: Prentice Hall, 1965.

Sussman, M.B. The family life of older people. In R.H. Binstock and E. Shanas (Eds.), *Handbook of aging and the social sciences*. New York: Van Nostrand Reinhold Co., 1976.

Sussman, M.B. Family, bureaucracy, and the elderly individual: An organizational-linkage perspective. In E. Shanas and M.B. Sussman (Eds.), *Family, bureaucracy, and the elderly*. Durham, North Carolina: Duke University Press, 1977.

Tolliver, L. Social and mental health needs of the aged. *American Psychologist*, 1983, *38*, 316-318.

Wershow, H.J. (Ed.). *Controversial issues in gerontology*. New York: Springer, 1981.

Wylie, M., & Austin, C. Policy foundations for case management: Consequences for the frail elderly. *Journal of Gerontological Social Work*, 1978, *1*, 7-17.

Zarit, S.H., Reever, K.E., & Bach-Peterson, J. Relatives of the impaired elderly: Correlates of feelings of burden. *The Gerontologist*, 1980, 20, 649-655.

From Hospital to Home Health Care: Who Goes There? A Descriptive Study of Elderly Users of Home Health Care Services Post Hospitalization

J. Dianne Garner, DSW

Although home health care services in the United States have been established sporadically since the Boston Dispensary started the first home care program in 1876, until recently this segment of the health care delivery system was largely ignored (Plass, 1978). With rising costs of health care, criticisms of institutional long-term care, and increased longevity resulting in increasing numbers of frail elderly, home health care has emerged as a partial solution to meeting the long-term care needs of the elderly.

The development and/or expansion of home health care services has received impetus from a number of factors: 1) home health care may prevent or delay institutionalization for some elderly (Kammerman & Kahn, 1976); 2) home care has been found to be the stated preference of the majority of elderly (Shannas & Maddox, 1976); 3) it is a way of expanding services and providing health care to an underserved population (Seidl et al., 1979); and 4) for some, it is a cost-effective method of delivering health care services (Oktay & Sheppard, 1978). In addition, there is a trend in recent national policy toward the position that health care needs of the elderly should be met first in the home with institutionalization offered only when care in the home is not feasible (Lowy, 1979).

Although there has been a marked growth in the professional literature around home health care in the past decade, there remains a dearth of descriptive information about the actual users of home

J. Dianne Garner, Director, Department of Social Service, St. Vincent Infirmary, #2 St. Vincent Circle, Little Rock, AR 72205-5499.

health care services. This article attempts to increase the body of knowledge regarding elderly users of home health care services focusing on those elderly entering home health care systems following acute-care hospitalization. Elderly users of home health care services post hospitalization will be described in terms of demographic data: age, sex, race, and marital status, and functional status at discharge from the acute care hospital. The following functional indices will be described: mental health status, behavioral impairments, impairments in activities of daily living, diagnoses, health status impairments, ability to manage medications, and communication impairments. Some comparisons will be made between the elderly discharged from the hospital into home health care and the elderly entering into nursing home care post hospitalization during the same time frame.

STRUCTURE OF THE STUDY

From May 15, 1982 through August 15, 1982, the Department of Social Service at St. Vincent Infirmary, a large acute-care general hospital located in Little Rock, Arkansas, gathered data regarding elderly users of post hospital home health services. During the three month time span, an assessment instrument devised by Arkansas Social Service, Arkansas Office on Aging, and the Arkansas Gerontology Center was used to insure uniform data collection. The population studied consisted of fifty hospitalized individuals 65 years of age and older who were referred to the hospital's Department of Social Service by physicians and discharged from the hospital into home health care. Concomitantly, data regarding forty-five patients 65 years of age and older discharged from the acute-care hospital into nursing home care was gathered for comparison purposes. The population studied was a 100% sample of patients meeting the stated criteria during the designated time frame. All data were gathered by ten professional hospital social workers and compiled by the director of the Department of Social Service.

LIMITATIONS OF THE STUDY

This study cannot be generalized to populations of elderly home health care users at large and no conclusions can be reached concerning elderly users entering home health care services from the community or other institutions such as nursing homes. Since hospital policy requires a physician's order for social work intervention, all elderly discharged from the hospital into home health care during the three month time span were not studied; rather, the study subjects were those hospitalized elderly identified as in need of social work assistance. Such identification within the hospital system generally implies one or any combination of the following: 1) there is a lack of familiarity with post hospital health care resources; 2) patient and/or family resources are limited; 3) there is difficulty making a decision regarding appropriate post hospital care; 4) the ability and/or willingness of the patient/family to follow through with post hospital care is suspect; 5) the patient is socially isolated; 6) multiple post-hospital services are indicated; or 7) initial social work intervention was requested in response to a problem unrelated to discharge planning. Given the procedure of referral for social work services within the hospital, generalization of findings of this study to all elderly users of posthospital home health care services should be approached with caution. A final limitation of this study is the relatively small number of the sample: N = 50.

DEMOGRAPHICS

Age:
Of the fifty patients studied who entered into home health care following acute care hospitalization, 21 (42%) were 65 to 74 years of age, 21 (42%) were 75 to 84 years of age, and 8 (16%) were 85 years of age or older. The actual age range was 65 to 97 years and the mean age was found to be 81 years (see Table 1).

TABLE 1

AGE OF POST HOSPITAL HOME HEALTH CARE

RECIPIENTS

AGE IN YEARS	NUMBER	PERCENT
65 - 74	21	42%
75 - 84	21	42%
85 and over	8	16%

Sex:

Of the 50 elderly recipients of post-hospital home health care services studied, the majority, 32 (64%) were female and 18 (36%) were male (see Table 2).

TABLE 2

SEX OF POST HOSPITAL HOME HEALTH CARE

RECIPIENTS

SEX	NUMBER	PERCENT
Female	32	64%
Male	18	36%

Race:

Of the 50 recipients of post-hospital home health care studied, the majority 34 (68%) were white and 16 (32%) were black. No other racial groups were represented in the sample population (see Table 3).

TABLE 3

RACIAL DISTRIBUTION OF POST HOSPITAL HOME

HEALTH CARE RECIPIENTS

RACE	NUMBER	PERCENT
White	34	68%
Black	16	32%

Marital Status:

Of the 50 recipients of post hospital home health care studied, the largest number, but not a majority, 24 (48%) were widowed followed by 15 (30%) who were married, 7 (14%) who were single, and 4 (8%) who were either separated or divorced. The vast majority, 70%, whether single, widowed, separated or divorced, were not married at the time home health care services were initiated (see Table 4).

TABLE 4

MARITAL STATUS OF ELDERLY POST HOSPITAL

HOME HEALTH CARE RECIPIENTS

MARITAL STATUS	NUMBER	PERCENT
Widowed	24	48%
Married	15	30%
Single	7	14%
Separated/Divorced	4	8%

In this study elderly post hospital home health care users were most likely to be widowed, white, females. No pattern of utilization related to age was demonstrated other than the drop in the number of users in the 85 and over age cohort. However, that drop may be as much related to the smaller number of individuals in the over 85 years of age group in the general population as to actual patterns of utilization of post hospital health care services.

FUNCTIONAL STATUS

Mental Status:

Mental health status was ascertained through utilization of a standardized ten point mental status examination administered by the hospital's social workers. Administration of the mental status examination prior to discharge from the acute care hospital revealed that of those elderly being discharged to home health care 42% exhibited clear mental health status, 24% demonstrated mild impairment in mental status, 24% demonstrated moderate mental status impairment, and 10% were severely impaired in mental status (see Table 5).

Behavioral Impairments:

Data related to behavioral impairments were gathered using three categories: 1. wandering, 2. abusive, aggressive, or disruptive, and 3. delusions or hallucinations. Of the 50 patients surveyed, 22 (44%) were found to have behavioral impairments and four patients

TABLE 5

MENTAL HEALTH STATUS OF POST HOSPITAL HOME HEALTH CARE

RECIPIENTS IN PERCENTAGES

CLEAR	MILDLY IMPAIRED	MODERATELY IMPAIRED	SEVERELY IMPAIRED
42%	24%	24%	10%

exhibited behavioral impairments in two separate categories. Behavioral impairments demonstrated by the sample population occurred in the following descending order of frequency: wandering = 12, abusive, aggressive or disruptive = 11, and patients exhibiting delusions or hallucinations = 3. The number of behavioral impairments was then collated by the degree of severity of the impairment: mild, moderate, or severe. The largest number of impairments, but not a majority, in all three behavioral categories was found to be mild, followed by moderate and severe (see Table 6).

TABLE 6

NUMBER OF BEHAVIORAL IMPAIRMENTS

BY DEGREE OF SEVERITY

DEGREE OF SEVERITY	WANDERING	ABUSIVE, AGRESSIVE, DISRUPTIVE	DELUSIONS/ HALLUCINATIONS	TOTAL
Mild	7	3	2	12
Moderate	5	6	0	11
Severe	0	2	1	3
TOTAL	12	11	3	26

A cross tabulation of behavioral impairments with mental health status revealed that all of the elderly individuals studied who exhibited behavioral impairments also demonstrated some degree of impairment in mental status, usually moderate or severe. However, the reverse was not true: regardless of the severity of mental status impairment, all elderly mentally impaired individuals being discharged to home health care did not demonstrate problem behavior.

Activities of Daily Living:

The activities of daily living assessed were bathing, dressing, toileting, continence, eating, and mobility. All elderly participants discharged from the hospital to home health care exhibited some impairment in activities of daily living. The average number of demonstrated impairments in ADL by severity was as follows: average number of mild impairments = 2.4, average number of moderate impairments = 1.0, average number of severe impairments = 1.8. The frequency of impairments in ADL occurred in the following descending order: bathing = 21, mobility = 17, dressing = 17, toileting = 13, continence = 10, and 9 patients demonstrated difficulties eating.

Health Status:

Participants discharged to home health care demonstrated an average number of 4.8 medical diagnoses. The most frequent medical diagnoses found were coronary disease, arthritis, organic brain syndrome, hypertension, stroke, diabetes, and cancer.

Health status was further evaluated in terms of the degree of functional impairment. Neither the number of diagnoses nor the diagnoses themselves were necessarily indicative of the severity of functional impairment. For example: one cancer patient might exhibit minimal functional impairment while another might be severely impaired. It was also found that elderly individuals with multiple diagnoses varied in functional limitations. Assessment of health status in terms of the degree of functional impairment produced the following picture of elderly individuals discharged from the hospital to home health care:

MILDLY IMPAIRED	MODERATELY IMPAIRED	SEVERELY IMPAIRED
4%	48%	48%

Medication Maintenance:

The need for assistance with medication administration and/or maintenance was assessed in terms of degree of assistance needed. Categories of needs were defined as follows:

—None—no medication or self-administered with no help needed.

—Low—monitoring or assistance needed less than weekly by caretaker.

—Moderate—professional monitoring or assistance needed less than weekly.

—High—regular or consistent professional monitoring and/or assistance needed.

Of the elderly individuals studied being discharged into home health care 18% demonstrated no need for assistance with medication, 25% demonstrated low need, 48% demonstrated moderate need, and 10% demonstrated a high need for assistance and/or monitoring of medications.

Communication Impairments:

Communication Impairments assessed included impairments in hearing, speech, and vision. The frequency of communication impairments in descending order occurred as follows: vision, hearing, speech. Communication impairments were additionally assessed by degree. For the elderly discharged to home health care, the average number of communication impairments by severity of impairment produced the following picture: mild = 0.8, moderate = 0.6, severe = 0.4.

A COMPARISON OF ELDERLY RECIPIENTS OF POST HOSPITAL HOME HEALTH CARE WITH ELDERLY RECIPIENTS OF POST HOSPITAL NURSING HOME CARE

Demographically, more elderly were discharged to home health care services in the 65-74 years of age category and to nursing homes in the 75-84 years of age category. Interestingly, for those 85 years of age and older, utilization of the two methods of post-hospital care considered (home health care and nursing home care) did not show a statistically significant difference. While females were the primary users of both methods of care, males were represented in the nursing home group slightly disproportionately to their numbers. Considering the racial representation of the populations sampled, no statistically significant difference by race was found among elderly users of home health care compared with elderly users of nursing home care post hospitalization. Widowed elderly were most likely to utilize both home health care and nursing home care followed by married, single and divorced or separated in descending order for both care options (see Table 7).

TABLE 7

COMPARISON OF DEMOGRAPHIC DATA

BY DISCHARGE OUTCOMES

DEMOGRAPHIC DATA		DISCHARGED TO HOME HEALTH CARE (N=50)		DISCHARGED TO NURSING HOME (N=45)	
		NUMBER	PERCENT	NUMBER	PERCENT
Age in Years:					
65 - 74		21	42%	12	27%
75 - 84		21	42%	25	56%
85 and over		8	16%	8	17%
	TOTAL	50	100%	45	100%
Sex:					
Male		17	34%	20	44%
Female		33	66%	25	56%
	TOTAL	50	100%	45	100%
Race:					
Black		17	34%	15	33%
White		33	66%	30	67%
	TOTAL	50	100%	45	100%
Marital Status:					
Married		16	32%	12	27%
Single		6	12%	3	7%
Widowed		23	46%	29	64%
Separated/divorced		5	10%	1	2%
	TOTAL	50	100%	45	100%

Mental health status was significantly more impaired for elderly recipients of nursing home care compared to recipients of home health care. While the home health care group was found to have a slightly higher average number of behavioral impairments than the nursing home group, the largest number of behavioral impairments of the home health care group were mild. The severity of impairments in ADL was greater among elderly patients discharged to nursing homes although the average number of impairments in ADL was the same for the two groups. Home health care recipients were most likely to need assistance with bathing; while nursing home recipients were most likely to be incontinent. Both groups demonstrated an average number of 4.8 medical diagnoses. However, of the participants discharged to nursing homes, 70% were found to have severely impaired health status compared to 48% of the participants discharged to home health care. Sixty-five percent of those elderly discharged to nursing homes had a high need for assistance with medication compared to 10% of the home health care group. Furthermore, nursing home care recipients were four times more likely to be receiving medication by injection than users of home health care services. Slightly more communication impairments were found in those elderly being discharged to nursing homes but both groups were most likely to have impaired vision.

SUMMARY AND CONCLUSIONS

Elderly participants in this study demonstrated multiple and complex difficulties indicating the need for well coordinated, multi-faceted home health care. Medically, the average number of diagnoses demonstrated was 4.8, and 48% of the population were severely impaired physically. In addition 58% demonstrated some impairment in mental status, 100% demonstrated one or more impairments in activities of daily living, and problem behavior was a common phenomenon. The vast majority of elderly users of post hospital home health care services (82%) demonstrated some need for assistance with administration and/or monitoring of medications. Communication impairments were common and ranged from mild hearing loss to total blindness. The fact that elderly users of post hospital nursing home care did exhibit more severe impairments than did elderly users of home health care appears to indicate appropriate utilization of the two care options studied and does not detract from the complexity of provision of home health care services.

The picture of post hospital users of home health care services presented by this study has multiple implications for social work practitioners in home health care agencies. Unfortunately, current Medicare guidelines severely restrict the number of reimbursable home visits social workers can make to home health care recipients. The home health practitioner in a limited number of visits (usually two) must attend to such tasks as, assessing patient and family needs, coordinating and arranging additional services, providing support to patients and care givers, while at times serving as a "watchdog" for possible abuse and/or neglect of elderly individuals who cannot attend to their own physical needs and who frequently exhibit behavioral and/or mental status impairments. Since care offered by the home health agency is generally time limited, the role of "discharge planner" from home health care is an appropriate social work role. Given the physical and functional status of patients entering home health care from the hospital as presented in this study, it would seem logical that home health practitioners as "discharge planners" will be involved in facilitating institutional care for some as well as assisting in making appropriate arrangements for continued home living for others. Awareness of the complexity of problems addressed by home health care social workers highlights the need for coordination between hospital social workers and practitioners in home health care.

From hospital to home health care: who goes there: the old, who in the face of multiple difficulties, choose to return home. Let us salute their strength and courage and those home health care workers whose skill, dedication, and very existence makes the choice possible.

REFERENCES

Kammerman, Sheila and Kahn, Alfred. *Social Services in the United States Policies and Programs*, Philadelphia: Temple University Press, 1976, pp. 237-386.

Lowy, Lewis. *Social Work with the Aging, The Challenge and Promise of Later Years*, New York: Harper & Row, 1979, pp. 127-133.

Oktay, Julianne and Sheppard, Francine. "Home Health Care for the Elderly." *Health & Social Work*, New York: N.A.S.W., 1978, *3* (3), pp. 39-41.

Plass, Penelope, "Home Care Services: How Many Can They Help?" *Health & Social Work*, New York: N.A.S.W., 1978, *3* (3), pp. 182-187.

Shannas, E. and Maddox, G.L. "Aging, Health and the Organization of Health Resources." *Handbook of Aging and the Social Sciences*, New York: Van Nostrand Reinhold, 1976, pp. 238-240.

A New Look at Home Care
and the Hospital Social Worker

Phillip E. Jacobs, PhD
Abraham Lurie, PhD

ABSTRACT. Clinical, administrative and social action reasons for expanding social work services in hospital based home care programs are persuasive. Hospital departments of social work should consider carefully how they may expand services in home care and coordinate and integrate such activities with social work and discharge planning processes occurring throughout the hospital. It is necessary for social work leadership to be present on professional advisory, quality assurance and similar committees and to use these committees as arenas for expanding the social work role in home care.

INTRODUCTION

In the past 15 years home care has emerged as a growth industry both in the for-profit and non-profit sectors of the health care industry. As modern technology lengthens the lifespan in general, and saves the lives of thousands of kidney, oncology, and heart patients who would have died fifteen or twenty years ago, society is faced with an increasing elderly and old-elderly segment of the population.

At the same time the revolutionary sexual, social and family changes that have occurred since the '60s have altered, probably permanently, the societal arrangements by which care of the elderly was provided formerly.

The Women's Movement, divorce, single parent families, working mothers and delayed and reduced child bearing have resulted in sweeping changes in our family life and how we care for our el-

Phillip E. Jacobs, Director of Social Work, The Long Island College Hospital, 354 Henry Street, Brooklyn, NY 11201. Abraham Lurie, Director of Social Work, Long Island Jewish-Hillside Medical Center, 270-0576th Avenue, New Hyde Park, NY 11042.

87

derly. The nuclear and extended multi-generational family which provided child care for our young and comfort, care and supervision for our old has become less and less common.

Given the interdependent nature of our social fabric, the freedom these dramatic changes have afforded many of us will have to be paid for in the coin of a new type of societal responsibility for the young and more to the point of this paper, the old and very old.

In addition to these societal changes, or more accurately because of these changes, the health care industry is also looking to home care to relieve it of a variety of burdens. As the percent of GNP spent on health care has soared to almost 10% of GNP[1] hospitals are being forced by the passage of legislation such as TEFRA and other acts of Congress to lower their lengths of stay, increase discharge planning effectiveness and lower the number of elderly patients who occupy acute care beds while awaiting transfer to nursing homes. The introduction of prospective reimbursement schemes, such as DRG's, further compels hospitals to do everything possible to discharge elderly patients who no longer require expensive acute care.

It is against this backdrop of social change and changes and reforms within the health care industry that the connection between hospital based home care programs and departments of social work attains greater importance. This paper focuses on three areas of interest: the clinical nature of social work services provided to home care programs, marketing and administrative issues related to social work services in hospital-based home care programs, and social policy implications relating to the growth of home care programs.

Clinical Issues

Oktay and Sheppard[2] outline the social worker's function in home health care programs as defined by the Federal Conditions of Participation as:

— Working with other members of the health team to assess the social and emotional factors related to the patient's health problems, and participating in the development of the patient care plan.
— Helping the patient and his family to understand, accept and follow medical recommendations and providing services that are planned to restore the patient to optimum social and health adjustment within his capacity.

—Assisting the patient and his family with personal, emotional, and environmental difficulties which predispose toward illness or interfere with obtaining maximum benefits from health care.

—Utilizing resources, such as family and community agencies, to assist the patient to resume life in the community and to learn to live within his maximum capacity.

—Participating in alternative and appropriate discharge planning.

In a paper on innovative roles for social workers in home care programs, Axelrod[3] identified the basic components of the social worker's role as casework, program coordination and planning. Axelrod pointed out that while social work services in this country had its origins in services provided to the client at home, during modern times there has been a shift towards providing help for the poor, the handicapped, the elderly and the psychiatrically impaired within institutional settings.

The renewed interest in providing social work services to the elderly in their homes has brought social workers back for another look at their roots. Social workers are "in their element" when servicing patients in their homes. While distinctions between social workers working in hospitals and others such as psychiatrists, psychologists, and counselors may be somewhat fuzzy, the difference between what social workers do in a home care situation as compared to the other members of the team is immediately apparent and clear.

For the chronically ill, the frail elderly, and the homebound, illness is not an event external to the fabric of their lives which requires primarily the application of specific medical technique or substance. This model of acute illness which responds easily and well to treatment, such as a tonsillectomy, or a simple leg fracture suffered by a thirty-year-old person, is the polar opposite of what a frail elderly person experiences when they are homebound due to COPD, diabetes, CHF, or cancer, to cite a few examples.[4]

For the chronically ill, frail elderly, homebound person, every aspect of life becomes affected and possibly changed as a result of the illness. Family relationships which may already have been strained, become more so. The patient not infrequently is pauperized by the cost of medical care, raising issues of self-worth, pride and dependency. Pre-existing personality problems can become exacerbated and feelings of anger, self-pity and hopelessness are common. Further compounding the problem is the frequent inability of the patient to perform simple activities of daily living such as eating, bathing and toileting.

The social workers become an indispensable part of the home care team. They are able to provide counseling, assist the patient with concrete financial, housing, and medical equipment problems, advocate for the patient with welfare, the health care system, Medicaid, support the patient in complying with the treatment regimes, help the patient understand and deal with strained family relationships and help the patient be reconciled to chronic illness. Indeed, in the absence of good social work care, home care services can be an exercise in the application of medical technology, while the patient remains miserable, kept alive physically but in turmoil and suffering emotionally.

Social work in home care, by providing services in the home, returns to the origins of the profession, to that subtle, artful blending of support, counseling and advocacy which social workers do best. Several examples illustrate the point:

L.Y. was a 79-year-old female who used to be a dancer and a domestic worker. She never married, and was living at the time of referral in a housing project. Her diagnoses included chronic alcoholism, CHF and diabetes. L.Y. was on Medicaid and Medicare, and had a worker at the local welfare office.

L.Y. was lonely, intermittently confused, agitated and depressed. She resented being homebound and wished to be more independent.

When visited by the home care social worker, the patient reluctantly divulged that her nieces, who also had drinking problems, regularly came to visit her when she received her checks. They would take her checks, leaving her a little money. They would go food shopping for her, but bought her salty canned foods, which were contraindicated for the patient.

Although she was malnourished, and impoverished as a result of her nieces exploiting her, she was reluctant to confront them as they were the only family she had, constituted her only visitors or link with the outside world, and did provide her with some food, however inappropriate.

The social worker helped the patient assert herself as worthy of not being exploited by her relatives. She held a meeting with the family members and the patient and helped the nieces to act more responsibly. With the consent of the patient, she worked towards arranging for the patient to have the checks directly deposited in her bank, with the nieces helping out by buying food that met the patient's dietary needs.

The different emergency situations in which a home care social worker is likely to become involved are shown by the following case:

B.A. was a 74-year-old bachelor at the time of referral. He had worked as a sailor in the navy, and as a merchant marine sailor, so he had an adequate income. Referred to the social worker for evaluation and planning, he had a history of several MI's and CHF. As the patient had never installed a telephone the worker made her visit unannounced. To her shock she found the patient to be in acute cardiac distress at the time of her visit. As there was no telephone with which to call for help, she sought the assistance of a neighbor to call for an ambulance which arrived promptly and took the patient to the hospital where he was successfully treated.

Upon his return, the social worker made several follow-up visits during which she convinced the patient to agree to having a telephone installed, which he could clearly afford. Complications with the phone company ensued as they had difficulty extracting the necessary credit information from the patient, who tended to be confused occasionally. In addition, they had difficulty in scheduling installation. The social worker intervened with the telephone company on behalf of the patient and succeeded in having a telephone installed in his home. Following this the patient felt more secure knowing he could call for help in the event of a medical emergency.

M.P. was a 64-year-old female who was a retired bookkeeper. Her husband, also in his 60s, was a former laborer who was on disability.

M.P. was referred for depression, apathy and a lack of progress in her rehabilitation. She was a diabetic whose leg was amputated and whose eyesight was failing. When first seen she was withdrawn, depressed and tearful. She acted as if she was hopelessly ill, and questioned the value of staying alive.

By counseling the patient and her spouse, the social worker was able to draw on the strengths of their relationship to support M.P. in her fight against her disabilities. Gradually her mood brightened, her interaction with her children and family increased, and her outlook improved. The social worker helped her obtain "talking books" from the library, and her overall use of leisure time improved.

The patient's improved affect made it easier for her husband to care for her, as he continued to assist her with toileting, cooking and bathing.

Administrative/Marketing Issues

Although inflation has cooled in most sectors of the economy, double-digit inflation still runs rampant in the health care industry. Because of this the Federal Government is insisting that hospitals cut costs in every way possible, including reducing the overall number of hospital beds and forcing more effective utilization of the remaining beds, requiring the elderly and poor to pay higher co-insurance costs, proposing to tax some health care benefits received by employees and making the first major change in reimbursement method in Medicare's history by shifting from a cost-based system to a fixed-payment system (the use of DRG's).

This intense scrutiny and tightening up of health care costs comes at a time of an unprecedented demand for health care services by the elderly. The National Institute of Aging predicts that by the year 2000 the population over 75 will have risen an unbelievable 53% since 1980.[5]

Taken together these two trends underline how crucial it will be for hospitals to discharge non-acute elderly patients as expeditiously as possible, indeed for many hospitals it will be a matter of survival. Hospitals and departments within hospitals, that are able to identify changes and new areas of service necessitated by the shifting social, demographic and fiscal context of health care for the remainder of the century will prosper.

What does this mean for hospital social work departments? Three things become apparent from this analysis. First, hospital social work departments will have to become more aware of the fiscal implications of their services, will have to build on their reputation as a caring, concerned group of professionals so as to include activities which help administration in their fiscal fight for survival. As Rosenberg[6] indicated they will have to work towards transforming themselves from "cost centers" which are cut in tough fiscal times, to "revenue centers" which are expanded and developed due to their importance. Second, they will need to demonstrate unequivocally how well-suited social workers are for discharge planning[7] and how much they can help hospitals to maximize the efficiency with which beds are used by helping to discharge patients as soon after the termination of their acute care as possible. With the implementation of a fixed-payment system of reimbursement, hospitals will simply no longer be paid for patients who stay beyond the reimbursable length of stay for their DRG. In this context, it is difficult to overestimate the importance of a good discharge planning department. It likely will spell the difference between fiscal solvency and bankruptcy (as it is meant to) for many institutions. Third, those departments and hospitals that exhibit a sensitivity to the elderly's needs will be more likely to attract this population group. By developing a philosophy that emphasizes the special needs of the elderly and frail elderly as they deal with the problems of chronic illness, departments of social work will be well-positioned to implement innovative programs for the elderly, be seen as a hospital resource on psychosocial problems of the elderly and generate additional revenue for the hospital through special programming. As hospitals re-align their services and priorities to deal with the elderly those social work departments which have already anticipated the emerging importance of this group to hospitals, by initiating or requesting programs that particularly benefit the elderly such as social work services in home care programs, will be in a better position to market their services to hospital administration.

Given these trends in health care financing and the growing importance of the elderly, we need as social workers to take a look at the administrative setting within which home care social work services are provided currently. At the present, home care departments are usually administered by nurses, usually with public health backgrounds.

Within the program, nurses frequently decide which patients will be interviewed by social workers, general criteria for referral, whether per diem or part or full time social workers will be used, and the extent to which the psychosocial needs of the patient should be interpreted to staff and stressed in the patient's overall care plan. Social work visits are not reimbursed unless the patient is receiving treatment as part of the overall nursing treatment plan.

Given the fundamental social changes in our society, and their implication for the elderly, is the time propitious to take a new look at the staffing patterns in home care programs particularly since the underlying problems causing the perturbation of the patient frequently are psychosocial as well as medical? Programs with "too much" medical emphasis and "not enough" psychosocial emphasis can end up dehumanizing home care patients by denying, avoiding and otherwise not adequately dealing with psychosocial problems.

This is an easy trap into which to fall in the home care field. As technology continues to extend life and provide technical fixes to medical problems, staff can become entranced by technology and forget that ultimately technology is a means to an end, rather than an end in itself. The goal of all technology is to restore health and a good quality of life to the patient. As those of us who work in this field know, how much easier to replace or repair the broken hip than to deal with the alcoholism or physical abuse which caused the injury in the first place!

It is the social work presence within home care programs that can help to re-focus staff energies and awareness on these psychosocial causes of medical problems. Social work can play a more important and significant role in home care programs, in several ways. First, the profession must lobby HCFA to alter the reimbursement regulations so that social work service be reimbursed as a freestanding service and social work services to patients' family members must be reimbursable as an essential part of home care social work services. Second, hospital social workers need to move into positions of leadership in home care programs. Given the medical sophistication of most experienced medical social workers, there is no reason why hospital social workers with management skills cannot play a more prominent role in the administration of home care programs. Third, home care social workers should not be restricted to servicing only patients referred, but should, in cooperation with the case managers and in consultation with other disciplines, be able to pick up home care cases on their own initiative as they do in most health care agencies. Fourth, the use of per-session or per-diem social workers in home care should be minimized in favor of social workers employed on a full-time basis within a hospital department of social work, whenever possible. Many home care programs currently use per-session social workers to make a home visit on a weekend or evening, and pay the worker an hourly fee for the visit. While an adequate type of service in most cases, this is not the most desirable way to provide service for several reasons. Quality social work supervision is difficult to provide to per-session workers, who in fact may never see a social work supervisor while providing per-session home care social work service. Workers on a per-session basis lack the opportunity to build up a specialized body of experience upon which to draw and grow from; their experiences tend to be isolated and fragmented. Per-sessions workers lack the informal learning experience of intermingling with their colleagues who deal with similar practice issues, and they tend to be isolated from the main hospital social work department. As a result, they don't have the occasion to attend departmental in-service sessions, workshops and seminars, and their professional growth is limited. From the social work department's perspective per-session workers are not available for participation in department-wide activities, such as service on departmental committees and task forces, and swing coverage for ill and vacationing workers, and as such don't provide the department with the depth of resources that a full-time worker does. Lastly, the use of a per-session social worker connotes a relatively unimportant, peripheral, clearly secondary role for social workers that is inappropriate, given the psychosocial nature of many of the problems of the chronically ill, homebound and elderly.

The process involved in hiring a full-time social worker in a hospital which had employed only per-diem social workers, illustrates several of the ideas expressed above:

> The hospital based home care program used several per-diem social workers to make home visits for those of the 700-800 patients who came on the home care program during the course of the year who were deemed to require social work help. The per-diem social workers received scant social work supervision, did not participate in any hospital social work activities and were unknown to the social work department. Approximately 190 visits per year to 130 patients were made by these workers, which clearly represented an underutilization of social work services.

With the cooperation of the Director of Home Care, a nurse, the decision to hire a full time home care social worker was taken. A candidate was selected who was acceptable both to the Director of Social Work, and Home Care and was hired.

The number of social work home visits increased significantly. The new social worker proved to be an asset to the hospital, since she was able to generate approximately more than her salary in Medicare billings.

The full-time social worker received full professional supervision from the Department of Social Work and participated in all departmental in-service sessions and committees. In addition to being able to help many more patients, she proved to be a valuable asset to nursing and other staff as she interpreted patients' psychosocial needs to staff within the context of their medical treatment. She became a valuable resource for the inpatient medical/surgical workers who consulted with her concerning home care patients readmitted to the hospital. In this way continuity of care between inpatient social work service and home care social work service was enhanced significantly.

As the potential for a hospital social work department's involvement in home care departments is realized, it will be possible to capitalize on outside funding and demonstration projects relating to home care. For example, in one hospital approval was obtained to participate in a home-care demonstration project funded by the local Hospital Association and City of New York. The program, called the Transition Community Placement Program (TCP), provides home care services up to 56 hours per week for non-Medicaid patients awaiting placement who would return home if they had a home attendant which they are unable to afford. This program seeks to demonstrate that a small ($50-$60 per day) expenditure for a home care aide can save $350 in acute care hospital Medicare bills. The social work department was able to advocate for the hospital's participation in this program in an informed, effective manner, due to its prior involvement and interest in home care.

Increasingly, similar programs will be available and probably will be more likely to go to those hospitals whose social work and/or discharge planning departments have been involved actively with home care departments.

Implications for Social Policy

From a social policy perspective, demographic changes, the women's movement and sexual revolution and changes in the allocation of our resources for health care all bear on how hospital social work departments should relate to home care departments. The coming growth of home care departments is one small necessary outcome of these many changes.

Hospital social workers are in a unique position because of training and experience to be part of an "early warning system" for the health care field concerning the coming importance of social programming for the chronically ill and frail elderly. The push for health care cost containment in the light of spiraling health care costs and the coming use of DRG's in combination with living arrangements that leave the elderly feeling more vulnerable and alone have clear social policy implications for the profession.

We have an obligation to advocate for those types of programs, such as social work services in hospital-based home care programs, which meet the changing needs of the elderly. We need to negotiate for this program in different contexts. First, we must convince the Federal Government to reimburse hospitals for home care social work services to family members and significant others, and to home care patients who are not active nursing care patients. Second, hospital administrators, physicians and nurses need to be educated concerning the importance of home care social work services. Third, home care administrators should be made aware of the vital importance of home care social work services as indeed should the social work networks.

Social workers need to rise to the challenge presented by those homebound chronically ill elderly persons who need help and support. The advocacy role for social work in discharge planning, as described by Lurie,[8] will thus be broadened to include home care.

CONCLUSION

Departments of social work in hospitals without home care departments should take the initiative in their hospitals by suggesting that administration consider the fiscal benefits of home care programs in general and billable social work activities within home care in particular. Social workers identified with the idea of promoting a home care program, work with nursing to make it a reality, and do everything possible to create a hospital based home care program which employs full-time social workers.

If a hospital already has a home care program the following should be considered: first there should be an attempt to begin changing the social work department's "image" from cost-center to revenue-center by initiating a breakdown of income generated by the home care social worker beyond that person's salary and fringe cost, the "profit" generated by that worker. If the home care department contracts out for social work services or uses only per-diem social workers it would be beneficial to show administration how much more revenue would be generated if there was a full-time social worker.

Social work departments should coordinate and integrate home care departments' social work activitiy with social work and discharge planning activity occurring throughout the hospital. By increasing the social work component in home care programs, departments come closer to reaching what Rosenberg[9] has called a "critical mass" of social work resources needed to provide basic social work services to a hospital with flexibility and the potential for growth. The home care social worker should be able to "pinch hit" for a medical or surgical social worker, if an emergency occurs and the need arises.

Social work leadership should be present on professional advisory, quality assurance, and similar committees, so as to be able to use the committees as an arena for expanding the social work role in home care.

Clinical, administrative and social action reasons for expanding social work services in hospital based home care programs exist, and are persuasive. For these reasons departments of social work should consider carefully how they may expand their services in home care.

FOOTNOTES

1. June, Levine, "Federal Impact–Yesterday, Today and Tomorrow," *The Coordinator*, 2 (May, 1983): 4-12.

2. Julianne S. Oktay and Francine Sheppard, "Home Health Care for the Elderly," *Health and Social Work*, 3 (August 1978): 34-47.

3. Terry B. Axelrod, "Innovative Roles for Social Workers in Home Care Programs," *Health and Social Work*, 3 (August, 1978): 49-66.

4. Mildred M. Malick, "The Impact of Severe Illness in the Individual and Family: An Overview," *Social Work in Health Care*, 5 (Winter, 1978): 117-128.

5. Michael Waldholz, "New Programs Seek to Care for the Aging in Their Own Homes," *Wall Street Journal*, 3/8/83.

6. Gary Rosenberg, "Concepts in the Financial Management of Hospital Social Work Departments," *Social Work in Health Care*, 5 (Spring, 1980): 287-97.

7. Abraham Lurie, "The Social Work Advocacy Role in Discharge Planning," *Social Work in Health Care*, 8 (Winter, 1982): 75-85.

8. Abraham Lurie. (Ibid).

9. Gary Rosenberg, presentation at the Society for Hospital Social Work Directors Conference, Minneapolis, Minnesota, April 1983.

Foster Family Care for Frail Elderly: A Cost-Effective Quality Care Alternative

Rita Vandivort, MSW
Gaile M. Kurren, MSW
Kathryn Braun, MPH

ABSTRACT. For the last 10 years, the development of cost-effective, community alternatives for chronically ill has been a serious concern of many service providers and policy-makers. The expanding of the elderly population has been well documented. In this state, projections show a need for an additional 1602 long-term care beds by the year 2000, almost double the current capacity. The state Medicaid Program is searching for ways to reduce the 50 million spent in 1982 for institutional long-term care. Already experiencing the shortage of long-term beds, hospitals have a chronic loss of revenue potential through the holding of non-acute patients in the hospital while waiting for a nursing home bed vacancy. At the 500 bed acute care hospital, 25-30 beds daily are occupied by nursing home wait-listed clients. The average waitlisted days per patient is 20.4.

In September 1979, the hospital's department of social work began foster family care for elderly persons eligible for nursing home care. Foster families are extensively screened and trained for the severely dependent clients. The social worker and registered nurse team are closely involved in placements, developing and implementing an individualized written treatment plan to assure the clients quality of care.

Data collected over the past three years clearly indicates that this setting provides cost-effective, quality care. Overall scoring on bathing, dressing, toileting, transfer, and continence, utilizing the KATZ Activity of Daily Living, shows that 71% of the clients improve after 3 months on placement. Although 45% of the clients are incontinent of bowel or urine at the time of placement, 33% make sig-

---

Rita Vandivort, Assistant Chief, Gaile M. Kurren, Chief, and Kathryn Braun, Research Specialist are with the Department of Social Work, Queen's Medical Center, P.O. Box 861, Honolulu, HI 96808.

The research component of this program is supported by a grant from the Henry J. Kaiser Family Foundation of Menlo Park, California.

nificant improvement to only occasional accidents. With 41% of the clients at placement requiring adaptive device and assistance for walking, 48% of the clients show functional improvements in walking.

Most significant for continued survival of this type of care, the total program cost is half the cost of institutional care for these elderly clients.

The paper will examine the multiple needs served through the program: the ill elderly person's need of a therapistic, caring environment; the hospital's need to curb loss of potential revenue; and the need of the Medicaid Program to contain costs. The paper also reviews client characteristics, foster family characteristics, quality assurance, and overall cost-effectiveness of the foster family model.

INTRODUCTION

As social work professionals, in the course of our daily work with people in need, we are in a prime position to identify gaps in social services. We see the holes in the alleged safety net, and we have responsibility to help generate community based programs tailored to meet local service needs. This becomes of particular importance during these times of decreasing federal participation in social services.

Hospital social workers are in a strategic spot to recognize service needs in health care. Providing solutions is a complex task and involves working both within the hospital and outside the institutional walls in the community.

This paper will examine the development and implementation of a foster family care program as an alternative to nursing homes for frail elderly people. We will describe the success of the program as it relates to three different objectives:

1. To provide a community based alternative to the frail elderly in need of nursing care.
2. To utilize acute care beds within the Queen's Medical Center more appropriately.
3. To provide more cost effective long-term care services within the state Medicaid program.

LITERATURE REVIEW

This review will divide the literature into three relevant areas: 1) description and evaluation of foster family programs for the elderly; 2) evaluation studies of home and community based care of the elderly; and 3) determination of criteria to measure quality in long-term care settings.

Steinhauer (1982) reviewed the concept of foster family and found the first researched program in Gheel, Belgium in 1250 for mental patients. Dorthea Dix promoted the idea in the United States in 1850 after visiting a program in Scotland. Massachusetts started an adult foster care program in 1885 and New York in 1935. The Veteran's Administration has practiced foster family placement of psychiatric patients since 1951.

Most states now have some form of adult foster care available to elderly, mentally retarded and/or mentally ill groups, but only 3 programs are known which specifically provide nursing home level care to frail elderly in a foster home setting. Massachusetts General in Boston and Johns Hopkins in Baltimore developed foster family programs in 1978 after which the Queen's based Community Care Program was modeled. After one year of operation, Oktay and Volland (1981) reported that Johns Hopkins program participants, foster families and natural families expressed a high degree of satisfaction with the program and that the cost of foster family care was lower than nursing home care. The Johns Hopkins program has conducted a random sample longitudinal study of the quality and cost of foster family care versus nursing home care. Further results from this research, funded by the Robert Woods Johnson Foundation, are expected soon.

In the second category, examining cost effectiveness of community sources, the GAO (1982) reviewed the research on the impacts of expanded home health care services and found evidence that individuals receiving expanded services lived longer and expressed more satisfaction with their lives. However, only in cases where expanded home health care services were a clear substitute for institutionalization was a cost savings realized.

Pennsylvania's Domiciliary Care Program was evaluated by Sherwood (1981) who found that for elderly participants, the experimental group scored higher on indicators of optimism and positivism, engaged in more social activities, expressed greater satisfaction with their living conditions, spent more days in the community and had lower costs than the control group of matched elderly persons residing out the service area.

Robertson et al. (1977) evaluated the cost effectiveness of a hospital based flexible respite program for families caring for severely disabled family members at home. The authors found that patients were maintained in the community with an average cost per patient per year of 80 acute hospital days, representing a cost savings over nursing home placement of these people. Relatives, health care workers, and elderly patients all expressed satisfaction with this care arrangement.

Skellie et al. (1982) studied the cost effectiveness of Georgia's Alternatives Health Services Project (AHS). Although not shown with statistical significance, the clients who utilized AHS as a substitute for nursing home placement had fewer institutional days, lived longer, and had somewhat lower costs than members of the equally eligible control group from whom the AHS services were withheld.

The third category concerns the criteria of quality of care and quality of life in long-term care settings. In a population of chronically ill and disabled patients who will never be "cured" or fully rehabilitated, quality of care and quality of life become synonymous (Kane, 1981; Linn, 1974). Criteria to judge quality include expressed satisfaction (George, 1980; Linn, 1982); continuity with people and things (Harel, 1981; Lowenthal, 1968; Kulys, 1978); belongingness (Tickle, 1981); emotional bonding (Goudy, 1981; Snow, 1982); locus of control in self versus others (Wolk, 1976); mental status (Ernst, 1977); behavior and affect (Moriwake, 1974; Gurel, 1972); improvement in activities of daily living (ADL) skills (Brook, 1977; Linn, 1977; Gresham, 1980; Plutchik, 1970); decrease in psychosomatic indicators of depression (Zemore, 1979); as well as longevity (Noelker, 1978); staff to patient ratios (Linn, 1977); number of admission to acute or long-term care facilities (Robertson, 1977) and adherence to prescribed therapeutic regimes (Donabedian, 1966).

PROGRAM MISSION

The current population of elders 65 years and over in Hawaii is estimated at 73,000 or 7.8% of the total State population, below the national average. However, in the last two decades, the age 65 + group has increased 51.7% or 2 1/2 times the national elderly growth rate. Only Arizona, Florida, and Nevada have had a higher rate of increase in the same period. In addition, people in Hawaii have a life expectancy second only to Sweden and the highest in the United States: 74 years for males and 77.9 for females. As a result, those persons 75 and older account for the most rapidly growing population segment. By the year 2000, the rate of increase in the 75+ age group is projected to be 142%.

The phenomenal growth rate of the elderly has prompted great concern among various public and private agencies in Hawaii especially because of the 18,000 elderly who are in the 75+ high risk age group. With a median income of $7,321, compared to the national average of $8,057, Hawaii's elderly population fare poorly in a state with a high cost of living. An estimated 25% of the total 60+ years population have yearly incomes below $5,000, compared with only 6% of persons under 60 years of age. The Hawaii State Department of Health's Health Surveillance data indicated that 14.7% or close to 13,000 of those 60 and older have significant limitations or are unable to carry on major activities. Approximately 22% of persons 75 years and older have severe limitations in daily living.

The difficulties of these high risk elderly are particularly apparent to the health care institutions, where they are represented as disproportionately high consumers of care. At Queen's Medical Center, a 500 bed acute care facility representing 33% of the Honolulu metropolitan beds, those persons over 65 years of age are 20% of the total patient group and use 30% of the total patient days. The higher total patient days belies the higher average length of stay for this group: 10.9 days for those 65+ while persons 14-64 years of age have an average length of stay of 6.3 days.

Often, the longer stays of elderly patients are due to inadequate or unavailable options for care when the patient is ready for discharge. Despite the higher incidence of extended families, Hawaii also has the nation's highest percentage of working women. Because of the absence of women as caretakers within the home, it is often difficult for an impaired elderly person to return home to family.

Concurrently, there exists a shortage of long-term care beds in the State. The Hawaii State Health Planning and Development Agency estimates that non-availability of skilled nursing beds cost the State $2,874,200 in 1979, as patients waited for long periods in expensive acute care beds.

The long nursing home waitlists, with losses in potential hospital revenue, was the impetus creating interest of administrators at Queen's to establish the Community Care Program within the hospital's Department of Social Work. Designed to serve those at the intermediate skilled nursing level, the three original objectives of foster family care were: first, to provide quality care to frail elderly with trained, case-managed foster families; secondly, to be a cost benefit to the Queen's Medical Center by reducing the nursing home waitlist; thirdly to provide the care at less total cost than would have resulted if the client was institutionalized.

The objective of having the Community Care Program be a cost effective alternative to nursing home placement was in recognition of the escalating costs of long-term care. Reflecting national trends, over 40% of the Hawaii Medicaid budget was being spent on nursing home care. Facing the anticipated large increases of elderly, especially the at risk 75 + group, Medicaid planners were alert to cost effective alternatives. Therefore, planning of the program included long-range plans for Medicaid funding.

PROGRAM STRUCTURE

There are four major activities to support quality foster family care: 1) foster family recruitment and selection; 2) foster family training; 3) client selection and matching to an appropriate foster family; 4) case management of foster family placements. The clinical staff is comprised of two masters level social workers and a registered nurse, functioning together as a team. The team model is crucial to blend the medical and social needs of the chronically ill elderly client.

Foster families are recruited from the community by advertising, media articles, and informal "word-of-mouth" reference from other foster families. Prospective families must submit information on family members, education and employment experience, housing arrangements, and any physical or medical problems in the family. The foster family must have a regular income and submit references. If the family appears acceptable, the social worker and nurse team will make a home visit to evaluate more completely the physical facilities, the family lifestyle, and the proximity to other community services. The entire house is evaluated and architectural barriers are documented. Also the types of ethnic foods served, pets, and the family recreational pattern are noted. The team further obtains information on what preferences they have for a client: will they handle incontinence; do they prefer male or female; will they prepare special diets, etc.

Based upon this information, the team decides whether the family is acceptable to become a foster family. Diversity in lifestyles and ethnic groups is encouraged. As our clients represent a variety of personalities and life choices, the pool of foster families should also reflect a diversity from which to choose. The staff encourages the family to be very honest about what type of person would best fit. The more we know, the more likely is a successful match to a client.

The accepted families are then required to successfully complete a family care training course developed by the Community Care Program. The training is specific and concrete about how to care for ill persons at home. Registered nurses, social workers, dieticians, and physical therapists teach the classes. The Family Care Training Manual outlines the course content and is used both as a training tool and as reference material for the family. The content of the training includes: roles and responsibilities of foster family caregivers, personal hygiene, exercise, body mechanics, digestion and elimination, home hazards and accident prevention, emergency assistance, medical follow-up, medication, infection control, signs of illness, vital signs, adaptive equipment for bedroom and bathroom, use of crutches, canes, walkers, braces, and wheelchairs, range of motion exercises, decubitus care, basic nutrition and special diets, mental confusion, losses in chronic illness, stresses in caregiving, death and dying, depression, and promoting a client's independence.

This training has proven so successful that it has also been completed by over 150 families caring for their own relatives as well as by community workers in gerontology. A family support group began three years ago at the request of those caring for their own relatives. Through the group the social worker and nurse are able to assist families in expressing conflict, enhance usage of available community resources, and learn new techniques of home care.

The elderly clients for foster family care are primarily drawn from the hospital's waitlist for nursing home placement. The clients predominantly have been at the intermediate nursing level, although a few skilled nursing clients have also been successfully cared for by a foster family, with the aid of home health agencies. The registered nurse reviews the medical record and discusses the client's condition with the floor nurses and the private physicians. Based on this information, the nurse completes the KATZ Activities of Daily Living Scale. The total score is converted to a monthly amount (range $450-$750) which determines the monthly foster family payment. If the nurse recommends that the client can be adequately cared for at home, the social worker interviews the patient to assess motivation for placement, financial resources, communication skills, family and/or friends involved, and the client's preferences in a family. Client may prefer no children or pets, or have rigid dietary likes/dislikes. Although relatively unusual in our tolerant multiethnic atmosphere, clients may have strong racial beliefs. These can strongly affect the outcome of placement and as such must be respected.

After the patient assessment is completed, the team discusses whether an appropriate foster family is available. Experience has shown that even extremely dependent clients, with severe urinary or bowel incontinence, mental confusion, and limited mobility, may be well cared for in foster families. Very demanding or critical clients can become family members, but the caregiver must have patience and the ability not to personalize or internalize the client's behavior. Clients who do not do well in foster family care include those prone to violence, those addicted to alcohol or other chemicals, and chronic wanderers.

The most frequent reason that a client is not placed is that the patient's own family prefers institutional placement. Often, the family feels guilty that another family can provide the care at home. The family finds it easier to justify why they are not caring for their own relatives if he is placed in an institutional setting which is so different from a home setting. As a result, 37% of foster family clients have no relatives in Hawaii, whereas only 8% of those admitted to a nursing home have no relatives.

The prospective client and the foster family selected by the team meet prior to placement. Relatives may also visit the foster family home before decisions are made. It indeed is magic to see clients and foster family discover shared past experiences or similar interests and outlooks. If both sides agree to foster family care, plans for discharge are made. The foster family receives specific instruction on the clients' needs, described in an individualized treatment plan done by the Program's nurse. A referral for home care services is made in cases where further short-term nursing or physical therapy followup is required (about 65% of the placements).

Once in placement, clients and foster families receive extensive attention from the staff. The first three months are crucial for the longevity of placement and the amount of bonding that ultimately occurs between client and family. The social worker uses facilitative techniques to defuse conflict and contract negotiation to stabilize frictional situations. The nurse monitors the physical care and may do further family education on nursing techniques. Home visits by the team are done at least monthly and the first home visit is within the week of discharge from the hospital. The team mediates with the physician and other community resources. Program evaluation questionnaires are completed in private with both the client and the foster family.

The underlying strategy of the staff is to encourage both the client and the family to discuss problems with the team. Repeatedly, it is stressed that to have a problem is not to be a "bad" caregiver or client. Similarly, because of the frail nature of our clients, the physical deterioration of clients may have nothing to do with inadequate care being rendered. And caregivers must avoid internalizing blame for the client's chronic medical conditions. The more open communication between staff, clients, and families, the more likely the genuine adoption of the elderly person into the family.

THE CARING UNIT: CLIENTS AND FOSTER FAMILIES

The Community Care Program has served 93 clients in the past four years. All clients share certain characteristics. The clients are determined to be in need of an intermediate nursing level of care and are facing long-term institutionalization. Clients must have multiple medical conditions and severe functional limitations in activities of daily living. The clients have all voluntarily chosen to live with a family.

In other ways, the elderly persons that are served reflect a diversity of backgrounds, personalities, and abilities. Reflecting the multi-ethnic Hawaiian society, 40% clients are Caucasian, 17% are Filipino, 14% are Hawaiian, 10% are Chinese, 10% are Japanese, with a few clients being Korean, Puerto Rican, Guamanian, and Black. This ethnic composition is similar to the ethnic distribution of ethnic groups in elderly persons going to a nursing home from the Queen's Medical Center. The age of clients is between 50 and 95 years of age, with an average age of 76. Thirty-seven percent of the clients have no relative while 13% have spouse and children, 25% have only children, and another 25% have a relative that is neither spouse or child. Approximately three-fourths of the clients are eligible for Medicaid if they were institutionalized. Sixty percent of the clients are female.

Examining the care needs of foster families clients reveals their frail and dependent nature. About forty percent of our clients are incontinent of bowel or bladder at the time of placement. Interestingly, only half of these clients are still incontinent three months later, because the caregivers are often successful with implementing a bowel or bladder schedule. A device and assistance in ambulation is required for 62% of clients. A few clients are totally unable to walk, using a wheelchair instead, but architectural barriers prevent more regular placement of such people. Almost all clients require supervision of medication (83%) and 75% of clients need special diets. Thirty-eight percent of the clients are significantly disoriented to person, place, and time.

The high level of care and caring on the part of the foster families to the clients is truly impressive. Primarily, the foster families are caregivers in their 30s or 40s with children at home (75%). Many express a desire to "adopt" an elderly person so their children can have a "grandpa." Other caregivers tell of positive esteem from caring for their own parents and a wish to care for another elderly person in need. Many have experiences as nurse aides in nursing homes and would like to provide the care at home. The monthly foster family payment allows some women to remain at home rather than work.

Predominantly, three ethnic groups are represented in foster families: Filipino (54%); Caucasian (29%), and Part-Hawaiian (14%). The notion of an extended family in these groups is helpful not only in recruiting families, but subsequently when caring for patients, as the caregiver usually has backup assistance from mothers, sisters, local "aunties." Despite persistent attempts, recruitment of Japanese and Chinese foster families has not been very productive. As Oriental families have a high incidence of both marriage partners being employed, few members are at home to provide the 24 hour care needed by foster clients. Regrettably, this currently limits the number of Oriental elderly persons that can be placed. Most of the current Oriental elderly are first generation in Hawaii and many are unable to communicate their needs in English, thereby precluding placement in many instances.

FISCAL SUPPORTS

The Community Care Program has drawn on many community resources during the demonstration phase. The total foster family payment is based upon the functional level of the client, varying between $450 to $750 monthly. The client retains $40 per month for personal expenses and contributes the remainder of his/her personal income to the foster family. Clients usually do not have sufficient resources to cover the foster family payment; the average client contribution is $379 per month. The Program assures that supplemental payments needed are paid to the foster family.

Private charitable foundations have provided the supplemental payments, contributing over $200,000 in the past four years. One foundation, the King's Daughters' Foundation, is committed to individual stipends to elderly persons and has provided $150,000 to support foster family care. The Queen's Medical Center has supported the four staff positions. A $175,000 three year grant from the Henry J. Kaiser Family Foundation of Menlo Park is funding a research evaluation comparing elderly clients in foster families with matched elderly being placed in nursing homes.

PROGRAM BENEFITS: CLIENTS, HOSPITAL, MEDICAID

Three major goals have guided the implementation and subsequent development of the Community Care Program: 1) to provide quality care to frail elderly persons; 2) to be a cost benefit to the Queen's Medical Center; 3) to be a cost-effective alternative to nursing home care. This section of the paper will measure the Program's performance against these standards.

In July 1982, the Community Care Program research staff compiled an item analysis of the modified KATZ ADL Scale used since the beginning of foster family care. Twenty-one past foster family clients had records of their ADL skills at discharge and at three months post-placement. Of clients in this retrospective study: over half improved in toileting (57%) and in transfer (52%); 48% improved in walking; 33% improved in continence and dressing; 38% improved in feeding; and 24% improved in bathing. Functional dependencies in the first six KATZ ADL items (bathing, dressing, toileting, transfer, continence, feeding) were compared at discharge and at three months in aggregate groups. At placement, 57% of the clients had 5 or 6 dependencies out of the six items; at three months, 28.5% of the clients had 5 or 6 dependencies. At placement, 33% of clients had 3 or 4 dependencies whereas 28.6% clients scored in this group at three months post placement. Only 9.6% of clients at placement scored dependent on 2 or less of the six items, at three months 42.8% of clients scored dependent in two or less items. Total ADL score improved for 71% of the clients in this retrospective study.

The prospective research evaluation in process compares foster family clients with those who were placed in nursing homes. Analysis on 15 pairs matched on age and total ADL score at discharge indicates significant improvements in foster family clients. At one year, 80% of the foster families clients showed improvement in total ADL score, with 60% of the nursing home clients showing such improvement. Again, at one year, 13% of foster family clients showed deterioration in total ADL score, with 33% of nursing home clients showing the deterioration in total ADL score. Utilizing a different prospective 15 pairs match on age and ADL at discharge, the three month post-placement shows the same trend comparison. Improvement in the six primary ADL measures was shown in 80% of foster family clients; such improvement was seen in 54% of nursing home clients. No change was seen in 20% of foster family clients and in 33% of nursing home clients. Deterioration was not seen in foster family clients at three months, whereas 13% of nursing home clients deteriorated in the six key ADL items. Although the sample size is too small to be significant, we anticipate such significance as the research sampling continues. The research evalution is also measuring bonding, depression, life satisfaction and locus of control. Such data clearly supports that clients receive at least equivalent, if not superior, care in foster families compared to nursing home care.

The research evaluation further indicates that the Community Care Program is a cost benefit to the hospital. Medicaid patients discharged into foster families spend significantly fewer ICF waitlisted days in the hospital. Over a six month period (September 1982 to February 1983), patients placed in foster family care average 18.4 waitlisted days while patients placed in nursing home average 48.4 waitlisted days. Reimbursement for one ICF day is conservatively estimated as $120 less than acute care day reimbursement. This represents an average gain of $45,000 per month in potential revenue to the Queen's Medical Center. Monthly clinical staff costs are about $5000 per month and we anticipate even this will be reimbursed by Medicaid.

The third goal, to be a cost savings to Medicaid by providing less expensive care than nursing home care, seems clearly met. In 1983, the State of Hawaii applied to the Health Care Financing Administration (HCFA) for a Home and Community-based Waiver to allow

Medicaid payment for services to the Community Care Program. The HCFA formula for cost-effectiveness included total Medicaid cost for SNF/ICF patients; total recipients; 9% annual increase in cost and recipients; average length of stay; and new bed construction at FY 82 prices. The average monthly cost of nursing home care was $1,555.50 whereas total average foster family care was $627 per month. Medicaid would realize a cost saving of $828.50 per month for each patient placed in foster family instead of nursing home. The cost saving in FY 84, serving 40 clients, is calculated to be $445,680; serving 50 in FY 85, a cost savings of $607,321; in FY 86 serving 60 clients, the Medicaid cost savings is projected to be $789,612. HCFA granted the waiver effective August 1, 1983. The Community Care Program is now negotiating a contract with Medicaid and State regulations to cover services is in process. The Medicaid payments will cover not only foster family payments (as personal care and homemaker services) but also the clinical staff services for case management.

CONCLUSION

On all measures, the Community Care Program has been demonstrated to be a useful approach to the provision of community based care to a vulnerable group of aged persons. It has, in addition, served important organizational and fiscal requirements of the Medical Center.

BIBLIOGRAPHY

Brook, Robert et al. Assessing the Quality of Medical Care Using Outcome Measures: An Overview of the Method in *Medical Care* Supplement, 1977.

Donabedian, Avedis et al. Quality, Cost, and Health: An Integrative Model in *Medical Care*, 1982, p. 975.

Ernst, Philip et al. Incidence of Mental Illness in the Aged: Unmasking the Effects of a Diagnosis of Chronic Brain Syndrome in *Journal of American Geriatrics Society*, 1977, p. 371.

George, Linda and Bearon, Lucille. *Quality of Life in Older Persons: Meaning and Measurement*, Human Science Press, NY 1980.

Goudy, Willis and Gondeau, John. Social Ties and Life Satisfaction: Another Evaluation in *Journal of Gerontological Social Work*, 1981, p. 35.

Gresham, Glen et al. ADL Status in Stroke: Relative Merits of Three Standard Indexes in *Archives of Physical Medicine and Rehabilitation*, 1980, p. 355.

Gurel, Lee et al. Physical and Mental Impairment of Function Evaluation in the Aged: The PAMIE Scale in *Journal of Gerontology*, 1972, p. 83.

Harel, Zev. Quality of Care, Congruence and Well-Being Among Institutionalized Aged, *The Gerontologist*, 1981, p. 523.

State of Hawaii-Department of Social Services and Housing-Long Term Care Channeling Demonstration Program. *Long Term Care for the Elderly-Report of the Long Term Care Planning Group*, Dec. 81.

State of Hawaii-Department of Social Services and Housing-Title XIX Statistical Reports 2082, FY 82.

Kane, Robert and Kane, Rosalie. *Assessing the Elderly: A Practical Guide to Measurement*, Lexington Books, Mass., 1981.

Kane, Rosàlie. Assuring Quality of Care and Quality of Life in Long Term Care in *Quality Review Bulletin*, 1981, p. 3.

Kulys, Regina and Tobin, Sheldon. Interpreting the Lack of Future Concerns Among the Elderly, *International Journal of Aging and Human Development*, 1980, p. 111.

Linn, Lawrence and Greenfield, Sheldon. Patient Suffering and Patient Satisfaction Among the Chronically Ill in *Medical Care*, 1982, p. 425.

Linn, Margaret. Predicting Quality of Patient Care in Nursing Homes in *The Gerontologist*, 1974, p. 225.

Linn, Margaret et al. Patient Outcomes as a Measure of Quality of Nursing Home Care in *American Journal of Public Health*, 1977, p. 337.

Lowenthal, M. and Haven, C. Interaction and Adaptation: Intimacy as a Critical Variable in *American Sociological Review*, 1968, p. 20.

Moriwaki, Sharon. The Affect Balance Scale: A Validity Study With Aged Samples in *Journal of Gerontology*, 1974, p. 73.

Noelker, Linda and Harel, Zev. Predictors of Well-Being and Survival Among Institutionalized Aged in *The Gerontologist*, 1978, p. 562.

Oktay, Julianna S. and Volland, Patricia. Community Care Program for the Elderly, *Health and Social work*, 1981 © NASW.

Plutchik, Robert et al. Reliability and Validity of a Scale for Assessing the Functioning of Geriatric Patients in *Journal of the American Geriatrics Society*, 1970, p. 491.

Robertson, Duncan et al. A Community-Based Continuing Care Program for the Elderly Disabled: An Evaluation of Planned Intermittent Hospital Readmission in *Journal of Gerontology*, 1977, p. 334.

Sherwood, Sylvia and Morris, John. *Pennsylvania's Domiciliary Care Pilot Program: A Digest of Key Findings Concerning Program Effectiveness and Operations*, HRCA (HHS 130-76-12), 1981.

Skellie, F. Albert et al. Cost-Effectiveness of Community Based Long Term Care: Current Finding of Georgia's Alternative Health Services Project in *American Journal of Public Health*, 1982, p. 353.

Snow, Robert and Crapo, Lawrence. Emotional Bondedness, Subjective Well-Being and Health in Elderly Medical Patients, *Journal of Gerontology*, 1982, p. 609.

Steinhauer, Marcia. Geriatric Foster Care: A Prototype Design and Implementation Issues in *The Gerontologist*, p. 293, 1982.

Tickle, Linda and Yerxa, Elizabeth. Need Satisfaction of Older Persons Living in the Community and in Institutions in *The American Journal of Occupational Therapy*, 1981, p. 644.

US GAO. *The Elderly Should Benefit from Expanded Home Health Care but Increasing these Services will not Insure Cost Reductions*, GAO/IPE-83-1, Dec. 7, 1982.

Wolk, Stephen and Teileen, Sharon. Psychological and Social Correlates of Life Satisfaction as a Function of Residential Constraint in *Journal of Gerontology*, 1976, p. 89.

Zemore, Robert and Eames, Nancy. Psychic and Somatic Symptoms of Depression Among Young Adults, Institutionalizing Aged and Non-Institutional Aged in *Journal of Gerontology*, 1979, p. 716.